'Out of a hundred [...] t
twenty who regula [...]
and as many as fo [...]
episodes of extreme [...]

In *Migraine and Headaches*, Dr Richard Petty discusses the problems faced by migraine and headache sufferers, looking at the latest medical research on the causes of such problems, especially the relationship between certain foods and migraines and headaches.

Not only does Dr Petty critically appraise the more conventional medical approaches, but he also discusses several new types of alternative medical therapies: acupuncture, homoeopathy, hypnosis, biofeedback and reflexology, all of which may help solve this problem.

With a list of self-help and information services in the final pages, this is definitely a book for the headache and migraine sufferers who would like to make their long suffering a thing of the past.

Dr Richard Petty was educated at London University where he obtained a degree in Medicine as well as a BSc degree in Physiology. He worked at the Neurobehavioral Research Center in Boston, USA, in 1976 where he became interested in patients with emotional and language disorders. As a Research Fellow in Neurology at the Princess Margaret Clinic he was personally involved with migraine and headache sufferers, which led him to treat his patients at the Charing Cross Hospital with medical acupuncture.

Dr Richard Petty has also taught both undergraduate and post-graduate level medicine and has published many articles on various medical subjects. He is currently Senior Registrar in General Medicine at the Northwick Park Hospital and the Clinical Research Centre at Harrow, and a member of the Research Council for Complementary Medicine.

RILEY BRANCH

Migraine & Headaches

Treating the Whole Person

Dr Richard Petty

London
UNWIN PAPERBACKS
Boston   Sydney   Wellington

First published by Unwin Paperbacks 1987

UNWIN® PAPERBACKS
A Division of Unwin Hyman Ltd
40 Museum Street, London WC1A 1LU, UK

Unwin Paperbacks
A Division of Unwin Hyman Ltd
Park Lane, Hemel Hempstead, Herts HP2 4TE, UK

Allen & Unwin Australia Pty Ltd,
8 Napier Street, North Sydney, NSW 2060, Australia

Unwin Paperbacks with the
Port Nicholson Press
PO Box 11–838 Wellington, New Zealand

British Library Cataloguing in Publication Data

Petty, Richard E.
  Migraine and headaches : treating the
  whole person.
  1. Headache—Treatment
  I. Title
  616'.0472   RC392
  ISBN 0–04–616032–9

Set in 10 on 11½ point Palatino by Grove Graphics, Tring
and printed in Great Britain by
Guernsey Press Co. Ltd, Guernsey, Channel Islands

Contents

Preface

Virtually everyone gets headaches. Only about 10 per cent of the population seem to be immune. For most of us they are just occasional nuisances, often being precipitated by stress, tiredness, or alcohol. In many of these mild cases, a period of rest or relaxation is all that is needed. Occasionally the headache is more persistent. Under these circumstances a simple pain killer or the use of one of the alternative methods may be required. These options are discussed in detail in this book.

For many people headaches are much more severe and debilitating. In the United Kingdom alone there are estimated to be at least 5 million people who regularly suffer from serious, recurrent headaches, and as many as 10 million more who simply put up with repeated episodes of sometimes extreme discomfort. It is important to realise that virtually all headaches can now be successfully treated, although different methods work for different people.

In the last few years there has been a reawakening of medical and scientific interest in the problem of headache, and a number of important advances have been made in understanding some of its causes, resulting in several effective new treatments. We shall be discussing the good and bad points of conventional medical therapies in some detail.

At the same time that medical knowledge about headache is progressing so fast, progressively more people are interested in alternative medical therapies. Every doctor has patients who have tried one or other of these methods of treatment, or else are thinking of doing so. A recent British survey indicated that the number of consultations with alternative practitioners is increasing at around 11 per cent per annum. It may seem strange that this should be happening just at the time that conventional medicine is becoming so much more effective at dealing with the problem of headache. There are several reasons why patients are going to alternative practitioners. It is partly because they feel that conventional medicine has failed them, and partly because of a general anxiety about the possibility of drug side-effects. There is another important factor, and this is that alternative practitioners give a particular kind of service which to many people is very appealing. There are many different types of alternative medical therapy, but they all have in common the idea that the only way to treat a patient is as a whole individual person with a body, mind and spirit. Therefore each treatment is tailor-made.

In this book we shall be discussing several types of alternative medical therapy in considerable detail, but we must emphasise that if you suffer with severe recurrent headaches, and especially if they are becoming worse, then you should discuss them with your doctor before embarking on a course of alternative treatment. The reason for this is that very occasionally headaches may be a sign of some more serious disease, and it is important to make sure that nothing unexpected is going on.

Very many people are anxious to know why they get headaches, and we are now discovering some of the causes underlying several types of headache. In the final section of this book we shall be discussing some of this research in detail.

My interest in headache was initially stimulated during the tenure of a research fellowship in the Princess Margaret Migraine Clinic at the Charing Cross Hospital in London. My research there was funded by the Migraine Trust, with additional financial support from the British Migraine Association, and I gratefully acknowledge the assistance of both these bodies, who have done so much to promote research into headache. My greatest debt, though, is to all those patients who have co-operated in various research projects over the years, and who ultimately asked me to write this book.

The case histories are all based on actual patients, but certain details have been changed in order to protect their anonymity.

R.P.
London 1985

MIGRAINE

AND

HEADACHES

CHAPTER ONE

What Is Headache?

All types of headache can be diagnosed according to specific criteria. The reason for making a diagnosis is that this guides the form of treatment which is administered, and gives some idea of the prognosis, or the long-term outcome of an illness.

Pamela was a vivacious 34-year-old blonde housewife, with three young children under the age of 6. Since her late teens she had regularly suffered with bad headaches. She was able to give a very clear description of these attacks. She usually knew that she was going to get a headache about twelve hours before it started. She would start to feel lethargic and depressed and sometimes would yawn uncontrollably. This continued until she suddenly developed flashing lights in front of her eyes. A loss of vision started over to one side and was followed by bright shimmering lights in the same area. This phase of the attack lasted for between 10 and 20 minutes, and then the headache would begin. It always started on one side of her head, as a severe throbbing pain. Almost immediately she would begin to feel sick, and she would usually vomit profusely after about an hour. As the headache developed she would find bright lights and noise quite intolerable, and would go off to a darkened room to lie down. In the past this had often been very helpful, but now with the young children it was usually not possible. The headache would drag on for up to two days before it gradually receded to leave her feeling totally drained. It was another day or two before she would feel totally recovered. The attacks typically occurred in the three days before each menstrual period, but now in addition she was getting at least one attack each week. She commented that she had been headache-free

1

during each of her pregnancies. For the first few years she had found that simple pain killers like aspirin or paracetamol had quickly controlled the symptoms, but now the headaches stubbornly persisted despite having tried a large number of different pills and potions. Pamela's general practitioner finally referred her to a migraine clinic and she was successfully treated with a combination of drugs and relaxation training. She was able to stop taking regular medications six months later, and when seen for a follow-up appointment after a year, she had only very occasional mild headaches which she could easily control herself.

Pamela gave a typical history of 'classical migraine'. She had generalised symptoms for some hours before the attack actually started. She then developed flashing lights or loss of part of her vision, which is called an aura, followed by a one-sided headache with nausea and vomiting. These features are alone sufficient to diagnose the classical type of migraine, but Pamela still underwent a full physical examination to ensure that there was no other explanation for the headaches. She also showed some other common symptoms. The headaches had almost invariably occurred before her menstrual periods, and the recent increase in the frequency and severity of the headaches had occurred with the stress of having to look after three very small children. In the majority of women with migraine, it vanishes if they become pregnant. It is extremely uncommon to see pregnant women suffering from migraine. Finally, her response to treatment showed that she had got herself stuck in a cycle of headaches. It is often the case that if someone is having a very large number of headaches, then the first priority is to break them out of this cycle of getting one headache after another. If this can be done, then subsequent treatment becomes very much easier.

There are actually several different kinds of migraine, but the classical type is much the easiest to recognise.

Susan was a 22-year-old shorthand typist. Her headaches had started six years earlier when she first started to take the oral contraceptive pill. Within two months of taking the pill she began to develop such severe headaches that she had to stop taking it. Although the headaches then became less serious, she continued to have regular episodes of headache every six or eight weeks, particularly when under stress at work. Each episode of headache would come on over a period of two or three hours, but she had no warning signs before the attacks. She did not experience any disturbances of her vision, but the headaches were always one-sided and associated with profuse vomiting. There had recently been some increase in the frequency and severity of the headaches since she had started working with a word processor visual display unit. Her mother had suffered with similar headaches for many years. Apart from these headaches, Susan often suffered with a dull generalised headache which would start during the morning, and gradually become worse until she went home in the evenings. She never had the second type of headache at weekends or while she was on holiday. Her work supervisor became concerned at the amount of time which Susan was losing from work and showed no sympathy at all with Susan's headaches. She finally saw her doctor about the headaches and was quickly and successfully treated.

Susan gives a typical history of 'common migraine'. It occurs in the population about five to ten times as commonly as the classical migraine which Pamela had. Sometimes both classical and common migraine occur in the same person. In common migraine there are no warning flashes of light in front of the eyes, but as before the headache is one-sided and associated with feelings of sickness or frank vomiting. As with all types of migraine it tends to run in families (we shall return to the point about the inheritance of migraine in Chapter Ten). It is very common indeed to meet patients whose migraine was either triggered or made worse by the oral contraceptive pill. Migraine is in any case about three times more common in women than it is in men, but there is no doubt that the pill is now an important cause of the complaint. It may unmask an inherited tendency to get migraine. If women develop migraine while taking the pill, then it may take many months for it to go away once the pill has been stopped, and about 10 per cent of women continue to suffer with headaches indefinitely. We shall have to return to this issue of the pill and migraine, but many doctors now advise against the pill if a woman has a history of migraine, and bad migraine sufferers are usually advised to stop the pill provided that some other effective contraceptive can be used.

Many migraine sufferers find that a change in their environment may cause more headaches. The commonest sort of environmental change is increased stress, but there are undoubtedly now also a few people who get headaches from working with visual display units. There has been a good deal of research on the whole question of the headache triggers, and we shall return to a detailed examination of this later in the book.

It is quite common for migraine sufferers to have more than one type of headache. Susan also had generalised headaches which came on during the day at work, and these were undoubtedly tension headaches. When using conventional medical treatment it is important to deal with each type of headache. The alternative practitioner who is trying to deal with the whole person does not bother very much with the different types of headache; he devises a form of treatment which will take in all the different complaints (we shall return to this several times when we discuss alternative medical treatments). The final point which comes out of Susan's case is the problem of definition of migraine. This is more than an academic medical problem. Many people have mild headaches which have been incorrectly diagnosed as migraine. So long as the headaches remain mild and infrequent, usually no harm is done by this misdiagnosis. But sometimes these people assume that all migraine is mild and inconsequential. Susan's supervisor thought that she had migraine herself, and could not understand why it was necessary for Susan to lose time from work with her headaches. Until you have had a proper migraine attack you can have no idea how dreadful they can be for some people. Migraine comes in all shapes and sizes, and it must be made clear that it is much more than just a headache. It is better to think of migraine as an illness which has many different symptoms, but the most common is headache. We have already mentioned that some people get flashing lights in front of the eyes, a dislike of bright lights or loud noises, and sickness. Still others get numbness or tingling in parts of the body before the attack or sometimes even difficulties with speech, or paralysis. Many get a variety of abdominal symptoms during the headache phase, including diarrhoea. Some people find that they pass large quantities of urine as the headache starts, and most complain of tenderness of the scalp. There are even a few unfortunates who faint with migraine attacks or have severe dizziness. There is a whole spectrum of migraine symptoms stretching from those who never get anything except the flashing lights in front of the eyes, to those who spend several days each week in bed, vomiting with severe headaches. In medical and scientific circles there is a great deal of discussion about how all these different symptoms should be classified, but a detailed discussion of this falls outside our immediate practical concern. The interested reader will find relevant references at the back of this book.

Migraine is the commonest form of severe recurrent headache, but there are many other types of headache which need to be properly diagnosed if the correct conventional treatment is to be given.

David was a 48-year-old shipping clerk. He had been suffering from headaches for very many years. He could remember having headaches at school, and over the years they had become gradually more persistent and severe. Several doctors had prescribed tablets for him, but none had done much good. At the time that he was seen, he gave a history of a generalised headache which occurred every day and which he described as a tight band around his head. Although it was always present, it did not stop him sleeping. He thought that it was perhaps slightly better when he was on holiday, but he could think of nothing else which either increased or decreased his pain. He had been diagnosed as suffering from tension headaches, but did not accept the diagnosis because he did not feel that he was tense. The diagnosis was confirmed, and he was treated with a combination of relaxation training and medications. He showed a marked improvement in the frequency and severity of his headaches, but continued to have mild headaches on two or three days each week.

Tension headaches are extremely common. Most of us get them from time to time. They are usually generalised headaches which typically start in the back of the neck and spread over the whole head, rather like a Roman helmet. Tension headache is actually not a good term, because it implies that it is a headache which occurs because you are tense. It is actually a headache associated with contraction in the muscles of the neck and head. Technically this is referred to as muscle tension. Stress is certainly the commonest cause of this type of headache, but it is far from being the only one. Some people are so good at burying stress that they may seem to be calm and relaxed on the outside, but inside there lurks a whirlpool of stress and anxiety. In these people, physical symptoms like headache may be the only clue as to what is going on inside them. In some folk, tension headaches may be triggered by a different mechanism. A particularly common one is posture. Typing and driving are two occupations which often lead people to spend long periods in just those odd positions which can lead to headaches, and both are also associated with stress. Simple measures like changing the position or height of a chair can sometimes work wonders.

Clinically, tension headache and migraine are usually quite distinct. However, as we have seen, both may occur in the same person, and recent research suggests that migraine and tension headache represent two ends of a spectrum of recurrent headaches. We shall discuss this further in Chapter Ten.

There is one fairly uncommon type of headache which we must mention briefly. This is called 'cluster headache' or 'migrainous neuralgia'. As the name implies, it is a form of headache which typically occurs in clusters or groups, usually at the same time of the year. For a long time it was thought that it was a type of migraine, but it is now clear that it is a separate condition.

Charles was a 34-year-old London taxi driver. He was a heavily built man, over 6 feet tall. He smoked 40–50 cigarettes each day, and consumed large quantities of alcohol when off duty. Each summer for the last five years he had experienced a bout of excruciatingly severe headaches. The cluster lasted for exactly six weeks. During this time he would have five or six headaches each day, each lasting for one hour. The pain was always on the same side of the head and came on very suddenly. During the attack, the eye and the nostril on the side of the pain would water profusely. The pain was so severe that during the attack he would often bang his head against the wall. He admitted that he had often felt suicidal. There was no family history of headaches, and he had previously been fit and healthy. The pain had not responded to any form of pain-killing medications. He was finally treated successfully with a drug which he took on a daily basis throughout the cluster.

Cluster headache is one of a small group of very severe headaches. It is remarkable in that it occurs almost exclusively in men, while migraine, as we have said, is very much commoner in women. It is even more surprising that these men are almost all very tall and smoke heavily. The pain of cluster headache is extremely severe, and there are certainly a few people who have committed suicide during a cluster. There are now treatments which are effective in the majority of these patients.

There are some people who have headaches that do not easily fit into these groupings, and in some cases there may be a strong psychological component. The pain is real enough, but we cannot find anything which might be causing physical problems in or around the head.

Jack was a 64-year-old retired carpenter. Some thirty years earlier he had struck his head after a fall from a ladder. Since that time he had suffered with persistent headaches, which had led to his early retirement from work at the age of 50. When asked about his headaches, he would simply say that he had a severe all-over pain that 'was killing him'. He would make this statement while showing no sign of any discomfort at all. He had drifted from one doctor and one hospital to another over a period of nearly a quarter of a century. He always refused to do anything to help himself and refused any treatment which was offered. He came a few times for follow-up appointments, but he and his most recent doctor finally agreed that there was little point in continuing to see him.

People do undoubtedly sometimes get headaches after head injuries. In most cases they stop after a few weeks or months. In Jack's case, the complaint of headache had become a central part of his make-up; his whole life revolved around his head. Probably the only form of treatment which would have helped him would have been psychiatric, and this he steadfastly refused. He was afraid that he would lose some essential part of himself.

We have so far concentrated on the common primary headaches. There are many people who get headaches secondary to some other illness.

Paul was a 16-year-old schoolboy. He had been experiencing headaches over his forehead for the last six months. An intelligent but unathletic boy, his school work had also been falling off. He was brought to the family doctor by his extremely anxious mother who was convinced that Paul must have a brain tumour. The doctor examined Paul in some detail and did not find any evidence of serious illness. The boy had denied having any visual problems but the doctor tested his vision anyway. Paul was very short-sighted. His headaches and schoolwork both improved dramatically after he started to wear spectacles.

Problems with the eyes are a common cause of headaches. Sometimes spectacles are needed, or a change in the way that someone reads or works. There are also some uncommon eye diseases, for instance, glaucoma in older people, which may need other forms of treatment. Many people suffer with headaches as a result of dental problems, sinusitis and ear disease. The first of these has caused great controversy in the last three years, and later we shall discuss the research into this.

The case of Paul brings up one other point. His mother feared that he had a brain tumour. She was normally a slightly anxious woman, but this fear had been planted in her mind after hearing of a neighbour who did have one. Brain tumours are an extremely rare cause of headache. Despite this, if the headache is in any way unusual, or becoming worse, then every doctor concentrates on excluding this diagnosis.

There is one other uncommon but important disease which may cause headache.

Sophie was a 61-year-old retired catering officer who was usually very fit and healthy. She went to her doctor with a one-week history of increasing headache over her right temple. She also found that her vision was beginning to blur, and she had weakness in her shoulders and thighs. She had lost 8 pounds in weight during the week. Her doctor found that she was extremely tender over the right temple and her muscles were weaker than he would have expected. He diagnosed temporal arteritis, prescribed treatment with corticosteroid medications and referred her for specialist advice.

Temporal arteritis is an uncommon disease which almost always occurs in people over the age of 50. It is an important condition for doctors to diagnose, because if left untreated it can lead to serious problems. The main reason for mentioning it at all is that it is one of the uncommon types of headache which must be treated with conventional medical therapy. We shall be spending a good deal of time discussing alternative medical treatments, but it is important that it should always be used with the full knowledge and approval of your normal doctor. Just occasionally someone's headache is caused by some disease like temporal arteritis, and then alternative therapy would be quite the wrong form of treatment.

We will now discuss some of the conventional medical approaches to treatment.

CHAPTER TWO

How to Treat It: The Conventional Approach

Virtually all patients with headache can be substantially improved, though there remains a small number for whom medical treatment appears to have little to offer. Conventional therapy cannot yet offer a complete or permanent cure for the primary headache types — migraine, tension headache or cluster headache. The reason why we cannot permanently cure these headaches is that we do not as yet understand enough about the underlying causes. As we shall discuss in the final chapter of this book, there is justification for thinking that we may soon know sufficient to be able to tackle the root causes of headache and perhaps to offer cures, but that is still in the future. So, let us see what we can do now.

Whatever the type of headache, whether it is just an occasional nuisance, or something which is causing a major interference with life, the first step is to try to establish what triggers it. If you take the problem to a doctor, he will start by taking a history and perhaps examining you. From this he will make a diagnosis based on the sort of criteria which we discussed in the last chapter. This is always an important first step because the treatment varies for different headaches. This process may also reveal what is triggering the headaches, and the first stage in any treatment programme will aim to remove these triggers if at all possible. Even if you do not want to consult a doctor about your headaches, then giving a little thought to the things which bring on the headaches may enable you to get on top of them without doing anything else.

We must stress that you should not overindulge in attempts at self-diagnosis. If in any doubt, or if you are worried about your headaches, then consult your doctor. In particular if they are becoming worse or occurring for no obvious reason then you should certainly not persist in personal efforts at treatment without first checking with your doctor.

The trigger factors are the circumstances which may precipitate a headache. It is important to stress that most headaches occur as the result of several factors — it may need two or three things to happen at the same time to provoke an episode. For instance, you may be a migraine sufferer who sometimes gets attacks if you are exposed to bright lights. If you look back you might discover that bright lights will only do this to you if you are also tired and hungry. Sometimes an apparent trigger may turn out to be no more than a coincidence, but it is usually fairly easy to sort out the real ones. Because it usually needs more than one factor to trigger a headache, it means that you are unlikely to find any single factor which always precipitates an attack. If 60 per cent of headache episodes follow one particular stimulus, then you have probably found a real trigger. It is quite common to find that trigger factors change with time. Some people have had migraine for twenty years without ever once getting an attack after alcohol, and then in middle age regularly develop attacks after even small quantities. On the other hand, it sometimes happens that the influence of certain triggers becomes less with time. It is a good idea to reassess the situation every year or two.

What are the common trigger factors? Well, there are very many, and we hear regularly of new ones. The most extensive work has been done on the factors which may precipitate migraine attacks. By far the commonest migraine trigger is stress and worry. In one study, 50 per cent of a random sample of patients had their first ever migraine attack during an emotionally charged period. Typically the attack develops as the stress builds up but sometimes it occurs in anticipation of something stressful. One often sees people who get Monday-morning migraine. It is sufficiently common that for many years it was taken as evidence that migraine attacks occur when someone is trying to avoid something unpleasant. A whole elaborate psychological theory of migraine was developed. The most likely explanation is though that stress induces a number of chemical changes in the body which between them are responsible for the attack. There is an intriguing phenomenon that occurs in some people — those who get attacks of migraine when the stress is turned off. These unfortunates successfully negotiate the stresses and strains of the week and are then struck by headaches at the weekend or on holiday.

Peter was a successful 42-year-old advertising executive. He worked twelve hours a day and travelled extensively. A self-made man, he had all the trappings of wealth, including a cottage in the country to which he went each weekend with his wife and children. He never had any health problems during the week, but over the last five years each weekend and most holidays had been ruined by severe attacks of migraine. They were classical attacks, ushered in by a visual aura on Saturday morning, and continuing with pain and vomiting until Sunday evening. He was treated with a programme of stress reduction during the week, combined with a regular preventive medication and did show considerable improvement. About once a month he continued to have weekend headaches, but they tended to be rather less severe.

This was a classic situation of headaches occurring when 'the heat was off'. It does illustrate another important point: with headache as with many other symptoms it is possible to become so convinced that some factor will set off an attack that you can almost think yourself into one. This was a major problem with Peter. It took some time to convince him that his weekend headaches were not inevitable. For this reason, we recommend that although you should try to establish whether there are any obvious things which trigger attacks, do not become obsessional about it. The whole point of doing this is so that you can avoid trouble, not so that you can gloomily predict that you are about to have an attack.

How to Treat It: The Conventional Approach

Careful attention to the details of Peter's problem suggested the solution. As with most stress-related headaches, we know from research that the important point is that there has to be some change in the body's stress level, which is referred to as the level of arousal. The key, then, was to try to flatten out this level of arousal so that it stopped bouncing up and down. Perhaps this could have been done by making Peter's weekends more stressful, but that would not have been wise since we know how damaging stress can be. Instead he was trained to deal with stress in a different way. This takes time, but virtually everyone can be taught how to do it. Successful treatment often does take both time and the involvement of several people. There is more and more stress in all our lives, but most of the time there is little that we can do about it. What we can do is to alter the way in which our bodies and minds respond to stress. In the chapters on alternative treatments we shall be discussing ways to do this.

A trigger which is related to stress is sleep. Some people wake from sleep with a migraine attack which has usually started during the dreaming phase. Lack of sleep is a potent migraine trigger. It is so common that if anyone is suffering from a lot of headaches it is a good idea to suggest a change in sleeping patterns. If at all possible, try to get to bed earlier and wake a little earlier in the morning. There are some people who get migraine attacks if they oversleep in the mornings. This is sometimes a cause of weekend headaches, if people have a lie-in on Saturday or Sunday mornings. This trigger can be easy to deal with. Either do not oversleep, or else arrange to wake at the normal weekday time and then just get up for a few minutes. You can then return to bed and sleep. A simple commonsense manoeuvre which has been successful in several cases.

Research indicates that migraine sufferers have a greater than average reaction to a given amount of stress. It was once thought that migraine patients were more obsessional or ambitious than other people, but this is not true. There is no such thing as a 'migraine personality'. Another related myth is that people with migraine are more intelligent than the rest of the population. Unfortunately this is also false. There have been some great people who did have migraine, including Charles

13

Darwin, Sigmund Freud and Thomas Jefferson, but it is no more than a coincidence that they had the illness.

In women there is often a close relationship between migraine and the phases of the menstrual cycle. About 60 per cent of women who suffer from migraine report that at least some of their attacks are linked to their cycles. Many women stop having migraine after the menopause, although it is usually impossible to predict if this is going to happen. It is obviously not possible to avoid the menstrual cycle, but there is evidence that some women who suffer with premenstrual headaches can be helped with either vitamin B6 (pyridoxine) or else with the compound Efamol which contains the oil of the Evening Primrose. These treatments are still somewhat controversial and we shall discuss them more fully in the chapter on alternative therapy.

A particularly important trigger is the oral contraceptive pill. As mentioned in Chapter One, there is no doubt that it is associated with an increased incidence of headaches, especially migraine. If the headaches are troublesome, then it is necessary to decide whether it is best to put up with them in exchange for a convenient and reliable form of contraception. Pill-taking women with a bad headache problem are normally advised to stop taking it if they can use a reasonable alternative form of contraception. There is a more serious matter to consider: classical migraine sufferers who take the pill are at an increased risk of developing a stroke from a blood clot in the brain. Most women these days take a low-dose pill, which does cause fewer headaches, but it is not yet known whether the risk of stroke is reduced with the low-dose pill.

Changes in the weather do occasionally precipitate migraine attacks. This is uncommon in the temperate areas of the world, but certainly does occur in those areas where there are hot dry winds. Evidence suggests that these winds, like the Santa Ana of California and the Foehn of Central Europe, exert their effect by producing changes in the ionisation of the atmosphere. Commoner than actual changes in the weather are headaches triggered by bright dazzling sunshine. People who find that they get attacks under these conditions are well advised to wear dark glasses whenever the sun is particularly bright. We have already mentioned the migraine attacks which some people get after exposure to visual display units. It is sometimes possible to reduce the incidence of attacks by slightly reducing the brightness of the screen, and looking away from the screen as often as possible. A final weather-related trigger is high altitude: some people get attacks when they are up mountains. The author began to suffer quite a severe attack while in the Himalayas at an altitude of only 12,000 feet. It responded to some of the alternative measures which we shall be discussing later in the book, and finally stopped on descending to a lower altitude.

Strenuous physical exertion will quite often precipitate attacks of headache. It has been known for many years that minor bumps on the head, for instance from heading a football, will give some people a migraine attack, but the exertion itself may be sufficient; it can be added to the catalogue of jogging-induced health problems. Many people who regularly get this problem find that taking a couple of aspirin or paracetamol before exercise will solve the problem. Others respond well to a drug known as indomethacin, which is used in the treatment of arthritis, but is only available on prescription.

You will notice that we have not so far said anything about food triggers. Many migraine sufferers do undoubtedly get migraine after eating certain foods, and we shall discuss this in great detail in later chapters. The usual advice is that if you are having a lot of migraine attacks then it is wise to remove certain foods from your diet for a trial period. The foods most often implicated in migraine are cheese, chocolate, citrus fruit, red wine and coffee. There is no evidence that these foods precipitate any other forms of headache, although other foods might possibly do so. In recent years there has been a lot of interest in the headaches precipitated by American hot dogs and those which follow Chinese food. In both cases it is a generalised headache which is caused by certain chemical additives — nitrates in hot dogs, and monosodium glutamate in Chinese cooking.

Naturally, you will not be able to avoid all the possible migraine triggers, but some knowledge of the things which may cause you trouble will help you to avoid some attacks of migraine.

What are the conventional treatments for headache?

First, before taking any medications, it is important to realise that whether or not stress was involved in triggering the attack, headache pain causes stress. It is easy for a vicious circle to be set up, in which pain causes stress which leads to more pain and then more stress. The other point is that headache, and migraine in particular, makes you very sensitive to sights and sounds around you. The smallest sound can become unbearable. The usual practice in headache clinics is to put the sufferer in a quiet, darkened room before doing anything else. If you can sleep, then many attacks of migraine will stop spontaneously. If you can possibly take yourself off somewhere and rest, it may do more good than any number of medications. These comments apply particularly to migraine, but the same approach is valuable with all headaches.

Most people will take a simple pain killer like aspirin or paracetamol. If this works then there is no need for any further action. Recently in Britain and in the United States, a drug called ibuprofen has become available over the counter without the need for a prescription. It has been used for many years in the treatment of arthritis, and it certainly does help some headaches as well. As with all powerful drugs, it does have a range of side-effects, although these are uncommon. It should not be taken by people with a history of allergy to aspirin, or of peptic ulcers, heart disease, or kidney disease. It should always be taken with food and stopped if it causes any gastric symptoms or heart-burn. This drug should also not be taken if you are on any other drugs, unless your doctor agrees. Another drug which is freely available is a combination called Migraleve. The author has rarely seen patients who found it to be of much use, but there is some evidence to show that it probably does help some people with relatively mild headaches.

In migraine, the problem of treatment is complicated because at the beginning of the attack the stomach stops working. This is part of the explanation for the nausea and sickness of the migraine attack. What it means is that drugs may not be absorbed. For this reason it is best to use soluble formulations of pain killers whenever possible. A relatively new but highly effective approach is to use drugs which combine a soluble pain killer with an agent which reduces nausea and vomiting, and gets the stomach working again. The two most widely used drugs of this type are Migravess, which contains aspirin and the drug metaclopramide, and Paramax, which combines paracetamol with metaclopramide. It is most important that any treatment must be taken as early as possible in the attack, preferably when the first warnings occur. It is much more difficult to treat an attack once it is under way.

There are various other drugs which are often used for treating the actual headache. Virtually all pain killers have been used at some time or other, and most are effective. In the last four or five years, a drug called mefenemic acid or Ponstan has been shown to be a very useful addition to the range of drugs which can be used in headache, and a recent research investigation has confirmed its value. There is a combination drug marketed under the name of Midrid (Midrin in the United States) which is little used, but is sometimes very effective in migraine.

One of the oldest drugs used in treating migraine is ergotamine. This compound exists in several different formulations. It comes originally from a fungus which grows on mouldy rye. Ergotamine is certainly an effective treatment for migraine and some cases of cluster headache, but it is ineffective in most other headache types. The trouble with ergotamine is that it is important not to exceed the stated dose, and it does leave many people feeling exhausted and nauseous for some time after the actual migraine attack has stopped. It can also not be used in people with a variety of different diseases, including peptic ulcers and heart disease. It is best reserved for people who get only very occasional attacks, and even then it is best used only when other measures have failed. A variant of ergotamine called dihydro-ergotamine (Dihydergot in the United Kingdom, D.H.E.45 in the United States) is effective in some patients, and appears to have fewer of the side-effects associated with ergotamine.

With this large range of medications, it is usually possible to find a drug which will at the very least give some relief. If the attacks of migraine are occurring frequently, then it is usually wise to consider regular treatment with the aim of preventing the attacks. All drugs and treatments have side-effects, and it is necessary to balance the risk of these against the pain and discomfort of regular migraine attacks. As a rule, preventive treatment is considered in anyone having more than two significant attacks of migraine a month. There is a lot of latitude in what constitute significant attacks and one tends to go on the amount of disruption which the attacks are causing. It is very common to see schoolchildren who start to get regular migraine attacks in the spring during the run-up to important examinations. They will often be offered daily treatment until the examinations have finished. It is usually better to do this rather than to jeopardise their exam performance.

Preventive treatment is administered each day, but as we said earlier, if you start on treatment it does not necessarily mean that you will need to take it indefinitely. It is often enough to use the drug to interrupt a cycle of headaches.

The most useful compounds for the prevention of migraine are certain members of a family of drugs known as the beta blockers. This has been clearly shown in several well-conducted clinical trials from Scandinavia, the United States and Great Britain. The beta blockers were invented during the 1960s for the treatment of high blood pressure and some heart diseases. It was purely by chance that these drugs were found to be of use in migraine prevention. The drugs of this class which have been shown to be most useful are propranolol, metoprolol and acebutolol. It is still a mystery why other drugs in this group are of little benefit.

Treatment with these drugs is usually started at a fairly low dose and then rapidly increased. It is sometimes necessary to juggle with the dose until the lowest effective dose is found. Most people with migraine happily tolerate quite high doses of these drugs without side-effects. The commonest of the side-effects are tiredness and cold hands and feet. They should not be used in patients with poor circulation or asthma. They are best avoided in diabetics, but interestingly diabetics suffer only rarely with migraine. As a general principle, it is important to avoid giving any drugs during pregnancy, but these drugs can be used if absolutely necessary. Fortunately it is very uncommon to have bad migraine in pregnancy. The beta blockers have a sustained benefit in over half the migraine patients who need to take it.

There are several other drugs which have been demonstrated to be useful in the prevention of migraine attacks. One such compound is the drug clonidine (Dixarit); in higher dosage this drug is sometimes used to treat high blood pressure. Clinical trials published in the early 1970s seemed to indicate that this was an effective compound, but later work has not confirmed this. The author has never found the drug to be of any use, although it is still widely prescribed.

The drug pizotifen (Sanomigran in the United Kingdom, B.C.-105 in the United States) has been used in migraine prevention for some years, and is certainly an effective drug for many sufferers. As with all the drugs used in migraine, it is not clear how it works but it does appear to alter the balance of certain key chemicals in the brain. The main side-effects of pizotifen are tiredness and weight gain. It stimulates the appetite in some people, and there are patients who have gained 20 pounds in the first month on treatment. It may be possible to avoid this particular side-effect by taking the drug in one dose at night.

The oldest of the preventive drugs is methysergide (Deseril). Related to the ergotamine drugs, it is very effective in many people, but it has been under rather a cloud because of side-effects. If used for long periods of time it has been associated with the formation of fibrous tissue in the abdomen. For this reason it is reserved for those patients who do not respond to other preventive drugs. It appears to be safe if it is given in interrupted courses of three or four months, with a one month gap in between.

One drug which is often effective, particularly if there is a lot of muscle tension associated with migraine, is the drug amitriptyline. This is usually used in the treatment of depression, but the effect in migraine appears distinct from its antidepressant action. It can often be combined with one of the other drugs like propranolol. Used in a low dose, it is sometimes a good treatment in people with tension headache. It does have a tendency to cause a dry mouth and constipation, but most of the side-effects of the drug do not occur when used at a low dosage.

In the early 1980s another class of drugs began to be used in migraine therapy. These are compounds known as calcium antagonists. They were developed for use in the cardiac pain known as angina, and more recently have been used for treating high blood pressure. The calcium antagonists have a number of varied effects on the body. As with the beta blockers which we discussed previously, this possible use for the drug was originally noticed by chance. There have now been a series of careful studies which indicate that some of these drugs, notably verapamil, flunarizine and nimodipine, may soon play an important role in the preventive treatment of migraine.

Several other drugs have been used over the years. Compounds like cyproheptadine, ergonovine and indoramin all seem to be effective in a few patients. During 1985, the first trials were published which show that another group of drugs may be valuable in the treatment of both the acute attacks of migraine, and to have a useful preventive action. These are drugs called 'Non-steroidal anti-inflammatories', or NSAI's for short. These are normally used for treating rheumatism and arthritis, and some are related chemically to ibuprofen which we mentioned earlier. The first of these to be shown to have this effect is naproxen. It is possible that other drugs in this group may be shown to have a useful effect in migraine, but we must await the results of trials which are currently under way.

This leads us to a final important point. Why is it that some people respond to one drug and not to another? Perhaps the major reason is that migraine constitutes a group of different disorders. All may seem the same from the clinical point of view, but the underlying imbalance varies among individuals. The other issue is that of placebo response. This is the response which people will have to any form of treatment, regardless of what it is. It is probably caused by a combination of psychological and physical factors. Placebo reactions may release a crucially important group of chemicals known as 'endorphins'. (See Chapter Ten.) Many sufferers are delighted when someone takes their illness seriously, and any new treatment which they are given will almost always be effective, at least for a week or two. Placebo reactions may muddy the waters when trying to establish whether a treatment is effective, but these reactions do tend to wear off with time.

We have an extensive and moderately effective armoury of drugs to use in the treatment of headaches. Careful attention to possible headache triggers will help many sufferers. It is often necessary to experiment with one or two drugs in order to find the best for the patient. Whichever drug is used, its value has to be balanced against any side-effects which it may cause.

CHAPTER THREE

An Introduction to Alternative and Drug-free Treatments

We have dealt so far with conventional, scientifically verified aspects of headache and its treatment, and turn now to the anecdotal and controversial. We should first ask the question: why is there so much interest in alternative medicine?

Even to those involved in it, the rate of progress in medical research is really staggering. It is estimated that the sum total of all medical knowledge is now doubling every seven years. Unfortunately, for the individual sufferer, research progress never seems to be fast enough. People want to be cured now rather than to be told that it should be possible to do more in a few years time. Until conventional medicine can deliver results that are safe and reliable, and treat the patient as a whole person, it is scarcely surprising that they continue to go to alternative practitioners, despite the poor scientific evidence that these therapies do any good.

All illnesses have both physical and mental components. Conventional medicine is becoming ever better at dealing with the physical side of disease, but it often seems that we are neglecting the mental side. Most doctors have always been acutely aware of the importance of dealing with the whole person, but constraints of time and money often make this difficult. Many patients also feel that if they go to see a conventional doctor, then they should come away with a prescription. It is by giving time, and by making it clear that they are looking at the whole person, that alternative practitioners score. The good deal of time which most will spend with the client will often do as much, if not more, than any form of therapy which they administer.

Alternative approaches to treatment have been around for a long time, and many have a history and tradition far longer than that of conventional medicine. They contain a number of different philosophies and techniques, and there is much disagreement between different schools of thought. What they all have in common is the idea that people consist of more than just a physical body. Therapy is aimed at the whole person, who is seen as a combination of mind, body and spirit. For most alternative practitioners this philosophy is inextricably linked to the methods which they use. It is seen as necessary to minister to all these parts of the person, and all alternative therapies stress the importance of the *will* to get better. They start from the point of view that all healing is really self-healing. Their role, then, is to help your body, mind and spirit to want to recover. This way of looking at people is very different from that of conventional medicine. It is important to realise that even the labels that medicine attaches to illnesses are not used by alternative practitioners. Since they are setting out to treat the whole of you, they work on the assumption that your headaches reflect some sort of bodily imbalance The doctor's diagnosis is rarely of much interest to them. They are far more interested in what they discover from you. Since they are setting out to deal with the whole of you, and not just your body, the treatment will be directed towards a number of factors which are specific to you as an individual. Different people who may seem to have the same type of headache may receive quite different treatments (we shall be returning to this several times in this and the following chapters).

People are going to alternative practitioners in ever-increasing numbers. There are many reasons for this, including anxieties about the possible side-effects of drugs, frustration with the failure of conventional treatment to give them relief, and a general feeling that they want to be seen as more than a malfunctioning body.

In the last chapter we mentioned the role of the placebo response. It is now very clear that placebos can have profound effects on the body, changing the secretion of some hormones and even altering some elements of the immune system. It is now known that some forms of alternative therapy do have a useful effect in headache, but it is still difficult to be sure that the therapies are any more than powerful placebos. As far as the individual is concerned this is perhaps not too important. The only concern is whether a treatment is going to be effective. It is, though, a major problem as far as research workers are concerned.

It is the belief of the author that the alternatives to conventional treatment should all be expected to produce research data to back their claims in the same way that medical scientists have to prove that a treatment works, and what sort of side-effects may occur. This will not be an easy task, but the first steps have been taken with the co-operation of doctors and alternative therapists. There are two reasons for making this demand. In the first place, it is only right that potential patients should know something about the track record of any therapy which they want to try. The other point is that if we were to prove that certain alternative therapies are effective, then there are thousands of therapists who could work alongside conventional doctors. The entire role of doctors would then change. They could spend time and resources on those things which they have been trained to do and leave the alternative practitioners to deal with the problems which do not require large investments of high-technology medicine. Similarly, if research shows that these techniques are no more than powerful placebos, then it is important that patients should know that this is the case. As we have said, placebo treatments can be very powerful and effective in some situations.

The alternative medical treatments are for the most part harmless. There have undoubtedly been cases of damage caused particularly by acupuncture and chiropractice, but these are uncommon. After all, conventional medicine also causes a good many problems, primarily from the unwanted effects of drugs. The more worrying problem is that the use of non-medical treatments may mask or cause a failure of diagnosis of a serious disease. This is very uncommon, but the author has seen one patient to whom this happened. It is important that the appropriate form of treatment is used. For this reason, if you decide to opt for any form of alternative medical treatment, then this must be done with the knowledge and consent of your own doctor. Over the last few years doctors have become very interested in the alternatives to conventional medical treatment. Most are now very receptive to the idea of their patients trying these different approaches. If they feel that they are not appropriate, they will usually say why.

If you do decide to consult an alternative practitioner, do make sure that he or she is properly trained. (We shall go into this in more detail in the individual chapters which follow, as well as at the end of the book.) There is a hope among both medical and lay practitioners that the introduction of stringent training requirements for all therapists will minimise the sort of problems which have sometimes occurred in the past, with unwanted side-effects and even injuries.

This leads us to the difficult question of whether you should only consult a medically qualified alternative practitioner. Perhaps in an ideal world all therapists should be medically qualified as well. However, because of the nature of their training, and sheer limitations of time, many doctors find it difficult to learn and practise alternative techniques. In addition, for the foreseeable future there will not be enough adequately trained doctors to deal with the demand, which will continue to rise, even in the absence of proof that these methods work. It is a reasonable compromise to say that alternative treatment should only be done under medical supervision.

There are well over a hundred forms of alternative medical treatment, and it would not be possible to deal with all of them in the detail which they demand. However, there are a number of excellent books available which will guide you through the finer points of these therapies. What we present here is the result of several years spent investigating a small number of therapies. This was not in any way a formal scientific evaluation, but one that was motivated by a desire to find out what, if anything, these approaches had to offer our patients; how they operated and how they approached problems. The following advice and discussion is the result of a good deal of time spent studying the therapies in question, and watching practitioners at work. This is not the conventional way to approach a problem in medicine or science, but it is important to realise that many major advances happened in just this way. Anecdotes were collected, and then formal scientific evaluations undertaken. Sometimes it turned out that there was nothing in the reports, but at other times simple but careful observation has revealed points of great importance.

It has become clear that the whole field contains a mass of contradictions and sometimes extravagant claims which can be very confusing to the potential client of these different approaches. We will try to show a way through this minefield, which will enable you to make an informed decision about what form of treatment you would like to try. A simple example will suffice. During these investigations, various practitioners declared that 90 per cent of all headaches were caused by dental problems, while others said that 90 per cent were caused by food sensitivity. There were also several other 90 per cents. It is very unlikely that all these claims are correct. To many practitioners of alternative therapies, the underlying philosophy of their methods is all important, but we have preferred to concentrate on results, in the belief that it is these that really interest the potential new client.

We shall return many times to the specifics of how often to have treatments, and how to judge if they are helping you, but at this point we can say that there are three rules if you decide to go in for alternative medical treatment:

1 Do it with the knowledge of your doctor.
2 Only go to a trained and registered practitioner.
3 If you do not feel some effect within two or three sessions then you are unlikely to benefit from a therapy.

CHAPTER FOUR

The Link Between Food and Headaches

Most forms of alternative medical practice are little discussed in conventional circles, but not so the role of food in triggering headaches. In the last five years there has been a sometimes heated debate on the subject. Some headache specialists consider that food never causes attacks, while others claim that the majority of migraine sufferers are food sensitive. The truth probably lies between these two extremes. There are undoubtedly many people who cease to have migraine attacks if they exclude certain foods from their diets, and food sensitivity is probably commoner in childhood migraine. In the chapter on treatment we discussed the triggering of migraine by certain foods rich in a particular chemical: cheese, chocolate, citrus fruit, red wine and coffee are implicated in something like 20 per cent of people who suffer with regular attacks of migraine. There does not seem to be any clear triggering of other types of headache by these foods. If you suffer with regular attacks of migraine it is well worth omitting these foods from your diet for a month or so to see if it makes any difference to the frequency and severity of your headaches. Naturally, if you get less than one attack per month then it would be necessary to stop these foods for longer to see if there is any effect. Food triggers are less likely to affect people who have only infrequent headaches. There are several reasons why these particular foods may be implicated in triggering some attacks of headache. All these foods do contain certain chemicals which may induce migraine

27

attacks. The other possibility is that some people have so convinced themselves that certain foods cause them trouble that they will literally trigger their own attacks; the food and what it contains are no more than incidental. The combination of the taste and consistency of a food, together with a fervent conviction that it may cause trouble is enough to give some people a headache. If a group of migraine sufferers with an apparent food trigger are examined scientifically, then only half of them get headaches if they are given their danger foods without being able to taste them.

Migraine triggering by cheese, chocolate, citrus fruit, red wine and coffee is an established fact. The only dispute is the frequency with which it occurs. What is far more controversial is the idea that a whole host of other foods may also trigger attacks of migraine in some individuals. Although it is by no means a new idea, in recent years this concept has attracted a good deal of attention from a few doctors, who are referred to as clinical ecologists. Some alternative practitioners have been applying the principle for a long time.

Food and chemical sensitivity has become known as 'Food allergy'. If someone has hay fever, they get the symptoms of a runny nose and streaming eyes when they are exposed to pollen. This is a definite allergy, and there may be measurable chemical changes in the blood which accompany an attack. These chemical changes become important when trying to decide whether or not someone actually has an allergy. People who are food sensitive do not usually get these chemical changes, so we are not dealing with an actual allergy. This distinction is of importance when trying to work out the best way of treating people.

If you think about it, it does seem strange that people might become sensitive to food. After all, we are exposed to it all our lives, and one would have thought that the design of the human body would prevent this sort of thing from happening. The intestines have indeed developed a remarkable system for protecting us from chemicals and foods which we eat. In some people these protective mechanisms do not function normally. Some chemical constituents of food slip through the defensive net and get into the body. Even this can usually be tolerated, but if we also have problems with the defence systems in other parts of our bodies, then we may be in trouble. Many people find that they become food sensitive at various times, particularly when they are run down. Some women only become food sensitive before their menstrual period. The following case demonstrated this well.

Diana was a 34-year-old waitress, married with three children. She had suffered with bad attacks of classical migraine for the last twelve years, with the attacks occurring only in the three days before each menstrual period. She typically experienced a feeling of lethargy and started to yawn uncontrollably. This phase lasted for about twelve hours, and then she would start to notice flashing lights to one side of her vision. Ten minutes later she would be in the throes of a severe attack of migrainous headache with vomiting and diarrhoea. The attack continued until her period started, when the headache would gradually recede. She had tried a number of different treatments but only ergotamine containing compounds helped her. These would give her some relief from the headache but often made the vomiting worse. She had lost all her headaches during her pregnancies. Both her mother and sister had similar headaches and both had noticed an association with their periods. Because of the problems with ergotamine, Diana was anxious to try some other approach to treatment. Close questioning revealed that she consumed a large amount of cheese and chocolate. These were excluded from her diet for the week before each menstrual period and she immediately noticed a reduction in the severity of her headaches. She tried various other dietary exclusions and found that several foods were apparently associated with her headaches. She decided to avoid fruit, alcohol and coffee, as well as bread and wheat-containing foodstuffs for the week before each period, and stopped having headaches completely.

It is important to stress that any action will reduce headaches in some people. It is quite possible that these elaborate dietary measures were having no more than a placebo effect, but the fact remains that Diana had been headache free for a year when last seen. She was able to eat anything she wanted except in the days before a period, when she apparently became highly sensitive to a range of different foods. Her sister tried a similar approach, and found that excluding similar but not identical foods had a useful effect in reducing her headaches. We do not know if her mother was also food sensitive, since she had stopped having migraine attacks after the menopause. The author has now seen several women who put themselves on completely bland diets for the days before a period, with good effect. It must be stressed that this approach does not work in everyone. Despite all manner of dietary manipulations and exclusions, some people continue to get headaches. Part of the reason is that, as we have mentioned in a different context, most headaches are the result of several factors conspiring together. We have discussed here the combination of food and hormones. A similar effect may occur with the oral contraceptive pill. The author knows of one person who experienced severe migraine attacks after starting to take it. She did not wish to stop and investigated the possibility of food triggers. She subsequently discovered that excluding eggs from her diet led to a complete cessation of attacks.

In some, the combination of hormones and stress may trigger the attack. While in others hormones alone, but with a strong genetic contribution, may be sufficient. Migraine does run in families, and a strong family history may make you more prone to any kind of trigger factor. It is both the chemical constituents of foods and the make-up of the person eating them which contribute to food sensitivity.

The clinical ecologist considers that the situation is rather more complicated than just removing things from the diet, in the hope that you will be lucky and find a headache trigger. He sees food sensitivity as more than just a chemical reaction to constituents of foods. Certain chemicals arrive in the body, and normally you adapt to them. If something happens, like a change in hormones, then your body may no longer be able to adapt, and you develop chronic symptoms. If you stop taking in the food or chemical, then your body may react with a whole new set of symptoms. Many clinical ecologists consider that if you have a craving for a particular food, then you may actually be sensitive to it. This becomes important when trying to establish whether someone is sensitive to a particular food.

Cheese, chocolate, citrus fruit, red wine and coffee are then generally accepted to cause headaches in some people, and it is well worth excluding them from your diet for a trial period. Despite the arguments about other food sensitivities, it is certainly worth a brief investigation to see if this is a contributory factor to your headaches. If you decide to examine this possibility, then it must be done very carefully. There is no point at all in going on endless special diets in the hope of curing your headaches. Food alone is not the cause, it is only one of the triggers. There are some practitioners who develop bizarre diets for their clients, and then keep changing them. This is in no one's best interests. If you do not discover a food trigger quickly, then it is unlikely that you have one. If you decide to continue with this approach, then you can go to a clinical ecologist, but ensure that you only seek the advice of a reputable practitioner. Do not go on with this approach unless you see a positive benefit rapidly.

It is important to emphasise that any form of special diet must be nutritionally sound. You must still get the right amounts of vitamins and minerals. The most extreme example of an unbalanced diet was one consisting of rice, lettuce and spring water; this was actually given to one person. Not only did it do nothing for the headaches, it caused weight loss, and would undoubtedly have had more serious consequences if it had not been stopped.

The first step is to keep a diary of your headaches for a short period of time. This must not be done obsessionally, but a record of when you get headaches and their relationship to events in your life may be invaluable. This is really only worth doing if you get regular headaches, but if you do, then make a note of when they occurred, what you were doing at the time, and what you had eaten during the preceding twenty-four hours. Record both the foods that you have eaten, and if you developed any particularly strong desires for a food. This may be a food which causes you trouble. Even if you are one of those individuals who suffers from food sensitivity, this may not reveal it, but it is a very good start.

To give you an idea how to proceed from here, it is useful to see how a clinical ecologist sets about the task of making a diagnosis of food sensitivity, and how he proceeds to treatment.

There are several methods of testing and treatment in use at the moment. It is easy to deal with people who can readily identify food triggers from a diary. If things are not so straightforward, then more sophisticated, specialised techniques may be needed. The most commonly used technique is the elimination diet. This starts with a five-day period when the patient is put on a fast. The idea of this is to cleanse the body of any harmful foods and chemicals which have already been ingested, and to make you more susceptible to any food which may be causing trouble. This is based on the idea that food sensitivity is like an addiction: stop taking an offending food to which your body has become adapted, and you first get withdrawal symptoms, and then, if you are exposed to it again, you get your original symptoms, but very pronounced. During this fast you are only allowed to take spring water. Some practitioners are rather less strict, and allow a diet of lamb and pears during this phase. These two foods rarely causing food sensitivity. It may be because lamb is less adulterated by chemical treatments than other meats, and pears are not exposed to as many chemicals as, for instance, apples and oranges.

Foods are then reintroduced one at a time, with each meal consisting of one food only. It is generally recommended that foods which you eat rarely should be introduced first. These are unlikely to be the cause of your headaches, and this method allows a more varied diet to be arrived at fairly quickly. You are then allowed to continue eating each food which has not caused any immediate symptoms. There is enormous variation in the list of foods which are said to be incriminated in headache, but some appear more often than others. Leaving aside the list of foods known to trigger migraine, in approximate order of frequency these are:

Nuts
Wheat
Corn or maize
Tomatoes
Milk and dairy produce
Yeast

It must be stressed that the clinical ecologist, although interested in the medical diagnosis, treats all headaches in this way, and claims that any may respond to exclusion of these foods.

It is said that the frequency of finding different foods which cause headache is related to the amount of the food which is eaten in the population. This is perhaps not surprising. If everybody eats cornflakes, but only one person in ten eats Chinese food, then on statistical grounds you would expect that more people are likely to get trouble from cornflakes. This is probably why the lists of headache-causing foods are different in books and scientific papers from Europe and from the United States; there are some substantial differences between American and European diets.

From various studies, it appears that people who are food sensitive are usually affected by more than one food at a time.

There are a number of methods for trying to establish whether someone is sensitive to a particular food. We have discussed the five-day fast, and this is used to see if you develop a headache after eating a meal. Although this sounds simple enough, there is often a considerable time-lag before symptoms occur. The fast is supposed to accelerate the development of symptoms, but it is not uncommon for a headache to develop up to twenty-four hours after exposure. It is then only possible to pin down the offending food or chemical if this is observed to happen on several occasions. For this reason, exclusion diets do seem to be a rather hit or miss way of tackling the problem, but it remains the easiest method for the individual to try. If you decide that you want to do this, then follow exactly the regime used by the clinical ecologist: the five-day fast followed by an ordered reintroduction of foods, one at a time. Naturally, if there are some foods which you never touch anyway, then it is not necessary to experiment with those. A word of warning though: do this at a time when there is nothing much else going on in your life. It is not feasible to go in for even a brief fast if you are working actively. Also do not contemplate this sort of approach if you know that you are a person who gets headaches when you are hungry. It is very unlikely that you also have a food sensitivity. If you develop a headache after eating a particular food, then you can treat it in the normal way with pain killers, or else by using one of the alternative methods which we discuss in this book.

Some clinical ecologists claim that you can reverse the immediate consequences of being exposed to a food by taking a mixture of sodium bicarbonate and potassium bicarbonate. The author has not seen this to be effective, but it certainly is a cheap and harmless treatment to try on yourself if you run into problems during the testing phase. Unfortunately this simple treatment does not seem to be of use in the treatment of headache at any other time.

Gillian was a 24-year-old unemployed secretary, who had suffered from typical attacks of common migraine for some years, and was now experiencing regular tension headaches. She had read about food sensitivity in a magazine, and was keen to discover if she suffered from it. The doctor who saw her was sceptical, but since she intended to pursue this anyway, he agreed to supervise the experiment. Gillian started with a strict five-day fast during which she only took spring water. She claimed to feel very well, although she had a minor headache on the second day. On the sixth day she had fresh orange juice and developed a headache two hours later. It was not as severe as the ones which she had experienced previously and it responded to some paracetamol. She had lamb and peas for lunch, without ill effects. In the evening she ate chicken and peas, again without problems. The following morning she tried some toast and was rewarded with a severe headache during the morning, which stayed with her for the remainder of the day. She felt too unwell to continue with the experiment on that day. On the next day she tried some breakfast cereal and again developed a headache. She carried on in this way for a week, during which she gradually reintroduced her normal diet. She found that she would reliably experience a headache after eating anything containing wheat or corn, including sausages and pies. She has now excluded these from her diet, and remains virtually headache-free. She has only very occasional attacks of migraine, and no longer suffers with the tension headaches.

It is said by clinical ecologists that just about all the chemicals in the environment may cause headaches in susceptible individuals. These include perfumes, petrol fumes, pesticides, and the fumes given off by gas cookers. The author has certainly seen a number of people who reported that they were sensitive to these agents. No one really knows if this type of sensitivity is common in headache, but it is clearly important to be on the look-out for agents like these which may be triggering attacks.

We have discussed the way in which you can approach this problem on your own. If you should decide to go to a clinical ecologist, there are several tests which may be used to see if you are sensitive to food or chemicals. They all try to get round the problem of the slow and somewhat unreliable approach of the fast followed by exposure to single foods. All these tests are still awaiting scientific validation, although they do seem to have been used successfully in some people.

The first of these which is in common use is the sublingual test. In this, tiny quantities of food extract are squirted under the tongue, and a record is kept of symptoms which develop during the test. At the same time the pulse is taken, because it is said that the pulse speeds up if you have just been exposed to a food which causes trouble. The pulse test is widely used but it seems unreliable and non-specific; the author has not yet been convinced that it has much value. The advantage of sublingual testing is that many foods can be tested in quick succession. It is doubtful whether it is particularly useful in headache, although it may be more valuable when trying to establish if certain foods are causing psychological symptoms.

Another test which is used by some practitioners is called intradermal testing. In this, food extracts are injected just under the skin. The places where the food is injected are then examined to see if a red wheal develops. If this reaction is seen, then it is thought that you are sensitive to the particular food. The quantities injected are miniscule and the test is virtually painless. Some clinical ecologists maintain that it is possible to use this approach for treatment, by injecting extremely dilute solutions of trigger foods. The idea is that you can be desensitised to these foods in the same way that some people with hay fever can be desensitised to pollen. This is an intriguing concept, and there do seem to be some people who have been successfully treated in this way. If you are sensitive to several foods, it can be difficult to organise an interesting diet. If this treatment works, it at least allows you to go back to eating anything you want.

A rather more respectable technique is the so-called RAST test, which stands for the Radio-allergosorbent test. It is designed to establish whether or not you have antibodies to certain foods in your blood. Antibodies normally exist to protect you against harmful agents in the environment, for instance bacteria. The idea is that if you have a food sensitivity, antibodies develop, and these are responsible for some of the symptoms. The test is in common use, but it is difficult to do it well, and there are a lot of questions about the relevance of the findings in individuals. Some people have positive tests to foods which have never given them a day's trouble, and others have persistently negative tests even when they are known to be food sensitive.

A number of other techniques for investigating food sensitivity have been developed in recent years. These include various types of electrical testing, and a method for measuring muscle tone after exposure to certain foods. These are most unorthodox and so far the author has not been convinced that any of them are of much use.

There is an urgent need to refine the diagnostic techniques used to detect food sensitivity. There is more and more evidence that clinical reactions to foods and chemicals are of great importance in medicine. It is also important to prove the point one way or another in individual patients. There are many people who are convinced that they have a food sensitivity, but when carefully examined they definitely do not. There are unfortunately a few people with major psychological problems who have taken refuge behind non-existent food sensitivities, and they have got the whole field of food sensitivity a bad reputation.

If a food sensitivity is recognised, there are three possible courses of action. You can avoid the offending foods for ever more; you can try desensitisation; or you can try a rotation diet. Rotation diets are also sometimes used for diagnostic purposes. The idea behind it is to eat a large variety of foods in a definite order, so you never get too much of any particular one. It is the repeated exposure to foods, on a daily basis, which is thought to underlie the development of food sensitivity. If your body has a break of a week before it has to deal with a particular food again, it reduces the chance that a food will ever cause you problems. For instance, many people are thought to get headaches from eating bread because they are exposed to it every day. If you only eat bread on one day of the week, it is far less likely to result in the development of a food sensitivity. During a rotation diet you are not allowed to eat anything at all more than once a week. The same approach can be used with foods which you know can cause trouble. If you have discovered that eggs cause you headaches, then limiting yourself to eggs only once a week may cause you to become immune to them. It is fairly easy to devise a rotation diet for yourself, and it is a logical extension of the exclusion diet. Again, this is a simple way of attacking the problem, but if you have not had a demonstrable effect within a month, then it is probably not worth continuing with this approach.

It is likely that food sensitivities cause chemical changes in the body. Another type of chemical change which may be responsible for many cases of headache, is hypoglycaemia, or low blood sugar. This is another controversial issue, with many denying the existence of the phenomenon, and others claiming that it is responsible for many different physical and mental symptoms. Your blood sugar is carefully maintained at the right level to allow the normal functioning of your body. In most people the mechanisms which are responsible for blood sugar control are extremely efficient; blood sugar varies very little during the day.

We have known for many years that patients who are being treated with insulin or tablets for diabetes may drop their blood sugar. If this happens they develop a whole constellation of symptoms, from sweating and palpitations to unconsciousness. Most physicians consider that it is only possible to drop your blood sugar level if you are taking these drugs; it is claimed that, except in a few rare diseases, the normal control mechanisms stop it happening at any other time. However, there are now a substantial number of cases of people who are not on any drugs, who have developed headache in association with a low blood sugar. Many of these have been successfully treated by a change in their diets.

Roy was a bespectacled 48-year-old educational psychologist. Successful and intelligent, he had for some years suffered with headaches and feelings of lethargy. The headaches always followed the same pattern. They would start during the morning, and would be gone by the afternoon. Often they would return in the early evening. In association with these headaches he would feel exhausted, have difficulty in concentrating, and his hands would often shake uncontrollably. The headaches were usually a dull ache above the eyes, but on occasion they would become quite severe, interfering with his work. It had been thought that these were simple tension headaches but they occurred just as frequently at weekends and on holiday. He was anxious to do something about the headaches and arranged for a full medical examination. This did not reveal any physical illness. Further questioning revealed that the headaches always stopped after he had eaten something. He smoked twenty cigarettes a day, drank a lot of strong black coffee, and usually had two large gin and tonics when he got home in the evenings. He was slightly over weight, and his diet contained a large amount of red meat, carbohydrates and fat. The symptoms sounded rather like those associated with drug-induced low blood sugar, but there was no obvious reason why he should be developing this. Although both he and his doctor were rather sceptical, his diet was totally reorganised. He was instructed to eat little and often, and to avoid refined (white) bread and sugar. He was also advised to stop drinking alcohol and coffee for a trial period. For general reasons of health he was advised to stop smoking. Within a matter of two weeks, he felt better than he had for many years, stopped having headaches and the episodes of shaking.

A doctor's usual reaction on hearing of this sort of case is to say that Roy's symptoms had nothing to do with the dietary manipulations; there must have been some other factor involved. Perhaps he was 'just neurotic'. Well possibly, but there is enough evidence to indicate that there are some people who do genuinely suffer from hypoglycaemia. Some practitioners, particularly in the United States, use a chemical test to help them diagnose this condition. This test relies on measuring blood sugar responses after taking a measured quantity of glucose on an empty stomach. It is an elaborate version of the test used in medicine to aid in the diagnosis of diabetes mellitus — sugar diabetes. Further work is needed to see if this test is as valuable as some people claim it to be. The idea that people on a 'normal' Western diet can develop a low blood sugar may seem strange. It is said that in people who suffer from this condition, blood sugar falls dramatically after ingesting the sort of foods which contain a lot of rapidly absorbed carbohydrate; it is a rebound effect. Taking large amounts of alcohol or rapidly absorbed carbohydrates causes the blood sugar to bounce up and down throughout the day and it is these rapid changes in blood sugar which may cause symptoms. At the moment, in the absence of definite proof that the glucose test is reliable, the best recommendation is to follow the advice given to Roy. If you have headaches which occur only at times when you are hungry and are associated with feelings of shakiness or sweating, then:

1 If you drink alcohol, cut down your consumption.
2 Eat little and often.
3 Avoid white sugar, white bread and white rice.
4 Cut down your consumption of sweet and fatty foods.
5 Eat more fibre and fresh fruits and vegetables.

Even if you do not suffer from hypoglycaemia, this represents an outline of the sort of diet which has many health benefits.

Having discussed the triggering of headaches by food sensitivity and by hypoglycaemia, we come now to a third type of dietary disorder which may be associated with headache in some people. This is the field of trace metal imbalance and vitamin deficiency. Vitamins and trace metals are closely associated together in the body, and so we deal with them together. This whole area is being actively explored by a number of distinguished doctors and scientists. Most members of the medical profession still regard the claims of these individuals as quite groundless, but there is evidence that headaches can sometimes be prevented by correcting these imbalances.

According to practitioners working in this field, several different vitamin deficiencies and trace metal imbalances may occur in chronic headache sufferers. Here we have a problem for the medical scientist. We have known for over a hundred years that there are certain illnesses that can be caused by vitamin deficiencies, and we can measure the levels of most vitamins in the blood. Routine measurements of vitamin levels have been done in headache sufferers, and these are usually normal. How then can we say that someone might be vitamin deficient in the face of a normal blood level? The answer, according to these practitioners, is that although you may have perfectly normal levels of the vitamin in your blood, the rest of your body may not have enough. Diagnosis and treatment are based on the clinical features of the headache: what it is like, and any accompanying symptoms.

The theory has developed that the body may need a big dose of a particular vitamin, both to restock the body and to correct imbalances between the different vitamins, as the balance between vitamins is regarded as being as important as individual deficiencies. The argument between practitioners of high-dose vitamin therapy and conventional doctors has raged for twenty years. Sceptics say that there is no point in taking vitamins for non-existent deficiencies, and in any case, only small amounts of vitamins are actually absorbed. Exactly the same set of arguments is used for and against trace metals in headache. They are difficult to measure and the interpretation of the results may be complex. A new and controversial technique for establishing the levels of metals in the body, is to measure them in a specimen of hair. Originally developed to measure the amounts of toxic metals in the body, some now also use the technique to measure the levels of trace metals in the body. This is claimed to give an accurate measurement, since the metals are incorporated into the hair as it grows. The method is not yet widely available, but if it can be shown that it tells us something useful, then we may hear a great deal more about it in the future.

Let us look at the claims of the practitioners and see if we can discover something useful.

The Link Between Food and Headaches

For centuries the navies of the world suffered the ravages of scurvy. In the 1740s, it was discovered that scurvy could be prevented by eating limes, yet it took some fifty years before the British Navy adopted the eating of limes as a policy and scurvy was wiped out at sea. Years later it was discovered that it is the vitamin C in limes which prevents the disease. Nowadays we rarely see scurvy in the Western world, except in the elderly or in the poor who are unable to afford to eat properly. The symptoms of scurvy are well known and most headache sufferers do not have them. Nevertheless, treatment with large doses of vitamin C (3,000 milligrams per day) has been said to be very beneficial in some patients. Is this just a placebo response or is there something more to it? Nobody has a definite answer to this question and we will have to await the results of clinical trials. In the interim you can investigate the possibility that vitamins may be involved in your headaches, without interfering with any other forms of treatment.

At several points in this chapter we recommend that you keep an adequate vitamin intake, but we must stress that you should not exceed the stated doses. In recent years there have been several reports of people who did themselves harm by taking enormous quantities of vitamins, and you must avoid doing this.

Many practitioners have stated that headaches may be caused by a mild deficiency of the vitamin B1, or thiamine. People deficient in this vitamin are said also to be irritable and depressed, to be apathetic and emotionally unstable. There can be many causes for all these symptoms, but some who have them do improve remarkably if they are treated with thiamine. Some doctors claim that drinking large amounts of coffee causes you to lose thiamine; perhaps this is why drinking excess coffee causes headaches and depression in some people. You may develop a chronic vitamin imbalance despite being on an apparently normal Western diet. Some foods may prevent the absorption of key vitamins, while others, like coffee, cause you to lose a vitamin in the urine. There may be a tie-up between headaches caused by the chemicals in coffee and headaches resulting from coffee-induced vitamin loss. The first of these is accepted by conventional medicine, and the second is regarded as being unorthodox.

Doctors who use high-dose vitamin therapy recommend that people deficient in the vitamin thiamine should take 500 milligrams of it twice a day for one week, and thereafter should stay on 50 milligrams each day. This dose will not do any harm but may do some good. The author has met a few patients who responded to this vitamin therapy. If you do decide to go in for the vitamin approach to treatment, it is probably best to take a combination of all the vitamins which we shall be mentioning here, and if you have had no effect within one month then there is no point in continuing.

A severe deficiency of the vitamin niacin (nicotinic acid) leads to the clinical condition known as 'pellagra', a complaint that is distressingly common amongst the starving and sometimes in the elderly, but rarely seen in the affluent West. Nonetheless, there are some who say that mild niacin deficiency does occur in many despite having an apparently normal diet. This milder type of the vitamin deficiency has many symptoms, the most important ones being headache and depression. The average daily requirement for niacin is around 20 milligrams for men and 15 milligrams for women. Normally you get ample in your diet by eating fish or poultry or brewer's yeast. When taken for headache or depression it is used in a dose of 50 milligrams twice a day, although there are some practitioners who use much higher doses than this. There are a few situations in which such high doses of niacin may be harmful, namely in diabetes, where it may elevate blood sugar, and in people being treated for high blood pressure in whom blood pressure may fall suddenly. If in doubt check with your doctor.

There is one final vitamin which has recently been extensively used in headache treatment. This is pyridoxine, or vitamin B6. Usually no more than about 3 milligrams of this vitamin is needed each day. As with the other vitamins, much higher doses are used for treatment. It has found particular use in dealing with premenstrual headache and premenstrual tension. The dosage for this is 150 milligrams per day.

Some years ago it was suggested that a number of different illnesses, including chronic headache, might be the result of a deficiency of various essential fatty acids. There was a good deal of dispute about this, but during this time a number of patients with headache were treated with the compound Efamol, which contains the oil of the Evening Primrose, a rich source of these fatty acids. It did not seem to be of much help to most headache sufferers, except those women who had premenstrual headaches. In some of these the improvement was dramatic and sustained. Nobody can accurately predict those who will respond to it, but a trial of Efamol is perhaps worthwhile in women with bad premenstrual headaches.

Several different trace metals have been said to be implicated in chronic headache. There is some dispute about the important ones even among alternative practitioners. The author knows of several patients who were treated with small amounts of the metal selenium. This was actually being given as part of an investigation into arthritis treatment, but some of the patients also had headaches, and reported that their headaches improved considerably. There certainly does seem to be a small number of headache sufferers who respond to this metal. Again, this may be no more than a placebo effect but it is the ultimate result which concerns us here.

Some practitioners say that headaches may result from 'poisoning' with certain metals — not trace metals these — but those that are found in the environment. Taking in small amounts of the metals mercury and cadmium may cause headaches in some people. These metals come from industrial pollution and cigarettes. The case for 'poisonous metals' is perhaps the most tenuous of all. There is no doubt that some people notice an improvement in their headaches if they stop smoking, but this could be for many reasons other than toxic metal exposure.

If you have headaches, and this approach to treatment appeals to you, then it is fairly easy to see if it might help you. Severe, sudden or worsening headaches are for your doctor, and not for these methods. Never overdo the vitamins and metals approach, and if you have not noticed a definite benefit within a short space of time, then there is little point in continuing.

First ensure that you are taking a sensible diet — we have already given you some pointers on this. Then, the experts would suggest, take the following high-dose vitamin schedule:

Vitamin C, 3,000 milligrams per day

Thiamine (vitamin B1), 500 milligrams twice a day for one
week followed by 50 milligrams each day

Pyridoxine (vitamin B6), 150 milligrams each day

Niacin, 50 milligrams twice each day

Most of these are available in combination tablets, and can be readily obtained from most pharmacists and health food stores. If you do have a beneficial effect from this regime then you can stop the vitamins after a month or two, and allow your diet to take over. This is a cookbook approach to using high-dose vitamins and those who use them in treatment tend to go for a more carefully devised regime for the individual. Nonetheless, this list will help many of you who are reading this. Do remember that there are dangers in taking too many vitamins, so do not exceed the amounts stated here.

CHAPTER FIVE

Acupuncture in the Treatment of Headache

Acupuncture is the best known of all the alternative therapies, and yet there has been more inaccurate information written about it than about any other.

In the West, it is practised by three groups of people. Medical doctors who have studied it at postgraduate courses, physiotherapists and some nurses, and finally lay acupuncturists. The training of lay acupuncturists varies enormously, from those who have undertaken full time training lasting several years to those who have only taken correspondence courses.

There are several different schools of thought about acupuncture. The main type which is available in the West is traditional Chinese acupuncture. This is a very ancient system, and acupuncture is only one part of traditional Chinese medicine (TCM). In recent years, in the West, a form of treatment has been developed in which needles are used, but in every other way it is quite different from the traditional Chinese form. This new system has come to be known as medical or scientific acupuncture. It deals primarily with symptoms, while the traditional approach aims to deal with the underlying causes of an illness. This new type is used mainly by some doctors and physiotherapists. If some part of you hurts, you may feel that rubbing the painful part relieves the discomfort. This is roughly what the medical acupuncturist aims for. He gently stimulates the tender areas, either with a needle alone, or else using a weak electric current as well. This can be a most effective way of dealing with many muscular aches and pains, and is often an excellent way of dealing with an acute attack of headache. It has also been used successfully for preventing attacks of headache. It is this medical form which has been subjected to the most research, but if you decide to have treatment with acupuncture, you are most likely to encounter a traditional practitioner. For this reason we shall concentrate on the traditional Chinese form of acupuncture.

Traditional Chinese medicine has been in use for thousands of years. The first records are at least 2,000 years old but there is some evidence that it has existed for much longer. Although it is typically associated with the Chinese, it has been found in more primitive forms in several parts of the world, for instance among the Eskimos. It is by no means a new import to the West; a few people have been using it in European hospitals for over 200 years. Totally different from Western medicine, it has its own complete system of anatomy, physiology and diagnosis. It relates illness to disturbances of energy in the body. In perfect health there is said to be a harmony between the basic forces called Yin and Yang. Everything in Nature is supposed to have two poles, like North and South, good and evil; one pole is always Yang while the other is Yin. Nothing can work unless these two poles exist and work together. The balance between these forces changes from day to day — we all know that on some days we feel better and more energetic than on others. In TCM, this is interpreted to mean that the balance of forces or energies in our bodies is varying from one day to the next. We shall deal further with the philosophical basis of TCM because this dictates how you are treated.

Apart from acupuncture, there are a number of therapies available within TCM, including herbal medicine, massage, nutrition, manipulation and the therapeutic exercises known as T'ai Chi Ch'uan. The practitioner sees it as his duty to deal with your basic complaint and then to keep you healthy in the future.

Gillian was a part-time accounts clerk in a large firm in the City of London. She had married ten years earlier at the age of

23 and had two children at primary school. She had suffered with headaches since her early teens, having attacks of classical migraine every ten days or so and also frequent episodes of tension headache. She had discovered many years earlier that cheese and chocolate sometimes caused headaches and had not eaten them since. Her doctor had tried a large number of different treatments over the years, and each had been successful for only a short time before she again returned to a regular cycle of headaches. She had read about acupuncture in a magazine article but felt a little sceptical that it could be of any help to her; she thought that she was too practical and 'down to earth' for something that seemed so bizarre. She was also put off by the thought of having needles stuck in her — it must surely be painful and might even be worse than her headaches. Also her doctor had treated her with great kindness and patience over the years and she was concerned that he would feel offended if she tried some alternative treatment. Worse still, he might refuse to have anything more to do with her in the future.

Then Gillian's headaches started to deteriorate again. She was losing time from work and found it difficult to look after the children. She felt that her husband was not being sympathetic and this made her situation even worse. Finally, she was prepared to try any treatment if there was a possibility that it might help. She discussed acupuncture with her doctor and to her surprise he supported the idea. She went to a practitioner who had a good reputation locally and had trained both in Britain and in China. She had a total of six treatments and to her surprise the treatment itself did not hurt at all. Immediately after the first treatment she experienced quite a severe headache but decided to continue with the course. In addition to acupuncture she was given massages by the practitioner, and several foods were excluded from her diet. The results were extraordinary: she stopped having headaches completely. Since then she has had one treatment every six months and has remained headache-free for two years. She is convinced that the improvement is entirely due to the treatment. Perhaps she has just responded to a sophisticated placebo, or perhaps the treatment has actually brought about some change in her, the nature of which we do not as yet fully understand. Whichever of these turns out to be the explanation, or even if it is a bit of both, the main point is that she has recovered.

In the West we regard people as made up of a collection of organs and cells which normally function together. Illness results if the various parts stop working in unison. In contrast, traditional Chinese medicine considers that the living person is a unity, and the idea of seeing people as lots of separate parts is just wrong. It is said that the vitality of any living thing depends on the uninterrupted flow of a life-force or energy called 'Qi' (pronounced 'Chee'). Qi is thought to flow around the body and is distributed by means of channels, which connect the internal organs together and also connect with the surface of the body. The internal organs are seen as performing all the functions accepted by conventional medicine, but in addition they have important affects on the mind and the emotions. The places where the channels come to the surface of the body are used for treatment by needling pressure, and are the so-called acupuncture points — the TCM practitioner sees the body covered in several hundred of these points. The lines or channels joining these points together are sometimes called the meridians. These are named according to their relationship to organs or systems in the body; for instance, there is a heart meridian and a liver meridian. In all there are twelve major meridians and eight minor ones. It has recently been claimed that it is possible to measure these energy channels electrically. Some practitioners claim to be able to see these channels running along the body.

The story of the discovery of the acupuncture points and the channels is largely shrouded in myth and mystery. There is no doubt that many of the main acupuncture points become tender when disease affects some part of the body, and it may have been this which gave the first clue to the existence of the points.

It is the flow and the balance of the vital energy, Qi, which is of crucial concern to the practitioner of TCM. There are said to be several types of Qi and headache is regarded as one of the manifestations of an imbalance between them. Imbalances of energy weaken the body and make it unable to resist the invasion of some outside agent. We might think in terms of a virus invading the body but the Chinese describe the invasion in terms of various types of weather. Fever, for instance, is described as a disease of heat, while the aching muscles which can happen with influenza are thought of as an invasion by wind. This whole way of looking at disease is, of course, very different from the conventional Western viewpoint, but a little reflection shows that there is at least some similarity between them.

If you consult a practitioner of TCM, the whole of the first part of the consultation will be spent trying to establish the nature of the energy imbalance. This requires great skill and experience but, as in any treatment system, accurate diagnosis is crucial if treatment is to be effective. The process invariably starts with a detailed history. At first this seems no different from the approach of the conventional doctor, but it soon becomes clear that the whole slant of the questions is different. The timing of symptoms is important — when exactly do you get headaches? What are the effects of weather, and of food? There will also be questions about the health of other members of your family. While you are answering the questions, and discussing your problem, the practitioner is listening not just to what you say but also to how you say it. Your expression, mood and speech are all regarded as being of crucial importance in helping him to decide on the exact nature of your problem, and how you need to be treated. This lengthy approach is all important because the treatment will be tailor-made for you.

After this comes a physical examination which is rather different from any that you are likely to have had elsewhere. If you have gone complaining of headaches, your head will be looked at, as well as any other parts which are causing pain or discomfort. The key parts to be examined are, however, the tongue and the pulse, and these are looked at in quite a different way from the conventional medical. Pulse diagnosis is a most important part of TCM. It is performed at the wrist. According to the Chinese you have a total of twelve different pulses which can be located at the wrist. There are three superficial and three deep pulses on each side, and each of these pulses relates to one of the organs or systems of the body. As we said, each organ also relates to a meridian or channel, so there are always the three things to be considered together: organ, channel and pulse.

Each of the pulses is examined carefully. The classical textbooks describe at least twelve possible variations of each pulse, so the possible combinations of pulse types are almost endless. For instance, you may have a rapid pulse which is wiry at the liver position but rolling at the spleen position; this combination means something quite specific to the traditional therapist.

There is nothing about these different pulses in standard Western medical textbooks, and in fact it is denied that they even exist. It is therefore most interesting that within the last four years there has been some preliminary scientific evidence to suggest that these pulses do actually exist. As pulse diagnosis is based upon centuries of careful observation, it would be amazing if there were nothing in it at all. Perhaps we have here yet another example of the West catching up with an established technique from the East.

We have described the classical way of doing pulse diagnosis. It is extremely difficult to do accurately and requires many years of experience. It is also a very time-consuming procedure — it is said that some classical practitioners would spend up to three hours just examining the pulse at the wrist. For this reason, a modified form of pulse diagnosis has been developed in China over the last few years. It starts with examining the pulse at the wrist, but instead of feeling at each of the twelve sites in detail, the aim is to get a general impression of the character of the pulse. It is decided whether it has deficient or excessive qualities, and this is taken to mean something about the state of the vital energy of the body. There is some recent evidence from China which suggests that this newer method of using pulse diagnosis is almost as accurate as the older technique, and so progressively more practitioners of TCM are now using it. It must be done in conjunction with an accurate history and the final parts of the examination — tongue and smell.

The use of smell is common in many different systems of diagnosis and treatment. This should not be too surprising; it has been known for centuries that certain diseases are associated with particular bodily smells. For instance, the uncontrolled diabetic may smell of acetone. However, the use of the tongue in diagnosis is particularly interesting. Although used to some extent in conventional medicine, the art of using the tongue to discover things about the working of the body has been developed to a very high degree in TCM. The tongue is again used, as is pulse and smell, to discover something about the balance of forces or energies in the body. The colour and character of the tongue are examined in detail, the coating of the tongue being regarded as highly important. Remember from our opening comments that the balance of forces, the Yin and Yang of Qi, alters from day to day. This means that the diagnosis which is arrived at will be different on different days. If treatment is to be successful, it has to be given so that it fits in with everything around you. Although you feel much the same on a Wednesday morning or on a Thursday afternoon, there will be subtle changes in you, and the good acupuncturist takes everything about you into account when he is planning your treatment.

After this sequence of diagnostic procedures, the acupuncturist is in a position to decide how he will treat you, basing his decision on a set of rules to decide exactly what to do. These rules are based on the traditional concept of the functions of the organs, and the relationships of the organs to each other. He may feel that the problem is one of an excess of heat or wind in the body, and there are particular points which are used to deal with this situation. Alternatively, there may be an excess of the Yang energy running along the liver channel, in which case this must be corrected. The whole point of treatment is to restore balance to the various energies, and thus to cure the body. There are specific points which are used either to sedate or stimulate different channels and organs.

Each of the rules that is used relates to a part of Chinese philosophy. The basic idea is that all things in Nature are interconnected, and time and number are regarded to be of fundamental importance. According to Chinese philosophy there are five elements — Earth, Fire, Metal, Water and Wood — and every organ in the body represents one of them. The liver is related to the element Wood, to the colour green, and the direction East. The heart is related to Fire, to the colour Red, and the South. There is a whole host of rules which can be applied but these examples at least suggest the complexity and sophistication of the system. Many of the rules and techniques are only taught to selected people, or are kept as carefully guarded secrets in families. These have not been recorded in any books and are only used by the most skilled and advanced practitioners of TCM. Despite all the rules and laws which govern the practice of TCM, ultimately the TCM practitioner, like any other kind of therapist, relies largely on his experience, carefully leavened by years of gaining the relevant knowledge. It is important to realise that the treatment you will receive will be quite different from that which will be given to anyone else.

These then are some of the general principles used by the TCM practitioner when he approaches a patient. Let us see how he tackles somebody with headache. We have made the point before that the alternative practitioner will invariably use a different diagnostic system from that which we discussed in the section on medical diagnosis. In theory, the number of headache types in TCM will be as many as there are patients, because everyone has a slightly different form of headache and the treatment will be carefully tailored to the individual. In practice, there are a relatively limited number of headache types encountered by most practitioners. People, although all individuals, do after all fit in to certain groups and classes. There are some fifty-seven common types of headache according to TCM. These are classified by location, by sensation, and by what is referred to as the 'internal condition'. There are at least seven different locations of headache, six different types of headache pain, and a large number of internal conditions which are thought to relate to the balance of energies within the body as a whole. There are specific recipes which can be used for dealing with each combination of symptoms, but they are always modified by any other findings which relate to the individual person.

What actually happens during the treatment itself? Many people are frightened or apprehensive about acupuncture because they think that it may hurt. Most of us have a few vague and unpleasant memories of painful injections in childhood, and these are enough to scare some people for life. In skilled hands, acupuncture is virtually painless. The needles used are considerably smaller than those commonly used either for giving injections or for taking blood. They also have a rounded rather than a cutting point, so they rarely cause damage or bruising and it is uncommon to draw blood. The needles are applied to various points on the surface of the body. The actual places where the needles are put is dictated by the findings of the diagnostic procedures — history, and examination of the body, pulse, tongue and smell. Many of the most commonly used points are located on the lower parts of the arms and legs. Sceptics have claimed that these points came to be used because the Chinese do not like removing their clothes, and these are the only parts of the body which you can get at. However, according to the underlying philosophy, the actual reason is that this is where the key points in the circulation of energy in the body can be located.

There is one other part of the body which is frequently used for acupuncture treatment — this is the ear. The development of a complete system of acupuncture applied to the ear is relatively recent. There are some references made to it in very old Chinese books, and it may even have been used in ancient Egypt, but much of its development has taken place in Europe over the last thirty years. It is based on the idea that on the outside of the ear there is a kind of map of the human body. This map represents all the organs of the body, with most of the skull and face mapped on the ear-lobe, the spine runs around the large inner ridge of the ear, and the hand somewhere near the top. In other alternative systems, it is said that the body is represented in the iris, or else on the sole of the foot. All these ideas seemed to be rather far-fetched, but then, in 1980, a scientific study was published which appears to give strong support to the idea of some sort of representation of the body on the ear. It was found that pain in various parts of the body caused the appearance of tender areas at specific points in the ear. Some practitioners in the West now specialise in the use of ear acupuncture, and the author has seen several patients who have been treated most effectively by this method. It might seem that having needles in the ear will be a painful experience but this is not normally the case.

When acupuncture needles are inserted, it is said that for maximum effect it is necessary to obtain a special sensation after the needle has been inserted. This is not the feeling of the needle going in, which many people do not feel anyway, but is instead a numb or dull sensation around it. It is rarely uncomfortable and people describe it differently. Some describe it as a tingling, and others as a feeling of warmth or gentle bursting. It is referred to as 'needling sensation', and it is obtained by gently moving the needle while it is in the skin. The sensation often moves up or down, and when it does this it follows one of the lines joining a group of acupuncture points. To someone with a medical training, the way in which these sensations sometimes move seems most odd. One particularly striking example was a patient who was treated at the beginning of an attack of migraine. One of the points selected was on the foot, at the third point on the liver channel. She immediately developed the needling sensation behind her eye on the same side. The treatment was successful but left something of a problem to the doctor. How to explain this movement of sensation? The patient knew nothing of acupuncture, so could not really have been making it up, and in any case similar things had been noticed before. The nervous system is the most complex piece of equipment known, but it obeys a number of rules. There are known pathways along which sensations run, and according to the current state of Western knowledge, there should be no such connection between the foot and the eye. Perhaps we will discover some sort of nervous connection in the future, but this phenomenon could easily be explained in terms of the channels. The liver channel starts in the foot and finishes up in the eye, exactly where this patient developed her needling sensation.

In order to obtain the needling sensation, and to alter slightly the effect on the point being treated, the needle will usually be gently moved after it has been inserted and you will be asked what you feel. Many therapists will take your pulse again during the treatment, and this will also guide any adjustments in the position of the needles. They are usually left in for between 10 and 20 minutes, and the number of needles used varies between four and about twenty. In China, it is often the practice to use far more needles than this, especially for treating severe or longstanding problems, but this is rarely done in the West. Sometimes the therapist also uses 'moxibustion' which is a technique of applying heat over an acupuncture point using the herb moxa. A compressed piece of this herb is stuck on the end of one of the acupuncture needles and lit, so that it smoulders. The smouldering herb warms the needle and is supposed to provide a certain form of energy to the acupuncture point and to the channel associated with it. In the East, people were often deliberately burned and scarred with moxa, but this is quite unnecessary and should never be done. Indeed, it is unlikely that there can be many practitioners in the West who use such drastic measures.

You now know something about what is entailed in having treatment with acupuncture. So the next question is, whether acupuncture or any other part of TCM likely to help someone with headaches? There have been several scientific trials which seem to suggest that acupuncture, both the traditional Chinese and the modern medical types, may help people with headaches. We cannot yet predict precisely which patients will benefit from this form of treatment, and for various technical reasons the trials will need to be re-done. Nonetheless, the evidence strongly supports the author's impression, based on several dozen cases, that acupuncture can be an effective technique both for treating acute headaches and for the prevention of headache attacks. If at the beginning of treatment you ask whether it is likely to help you, the practitioner will have to say that he cannot tell at that stage. After the first treatment he should be developing a fairly good understanding of you, and he should be able to give you some idea of your chances of improvement. A few people do respond almost magically to only one treatment, but this is unusual. If you do not feel any different after three treatments, then it is probably not worth continuing, but if you do, then you may need as many as a dozen treatments. Everybody is different in their response and in the number of treatments they need.

If the treatment seems to be working, then how often should you have it? This varies, but the average is once a week. The Chinese traditionally used very frequent treatments, sometimes several times in a day, but this is only rarely necessary. Many people show their greatest response to treatment in the hours and days afterwards, and so the gap of a few days can make it easier to gauge the progress of the treatment. Sometimes it is necessary to have another few treatments after a month or two, but the individual therapist will be able to advise about this. Some traditional practitioners will also give you some herbs to continue taking from time to time. We still know very little about these herbs but they may well contain some form of active chemical compound. It is worth bearing in mind that one European herb, Feverfew (Tanacetum parthenium), has been used in migrainous headaches for the last 300 years, but it was not scientifically proven until 1985 that it could be an effective treatment in some migraine sufferers. Feverfew is now widely available from herbalists and some health food shops, and many people are reporting its effectiveness. So long as a herb does not cause harm, there is no need at all for the headache sufferer to await the results of a scientific trial, if experience shows that it may do some good. Naturally the use of untested compounds in the treatment of serious or life-threatening conditions would be quite a different matter.

Some TCM practitioners also use a form of massage based upon the acupuncture points and channels. This may be used during the treatment session itself, or else in the time between treatments. Massage of any type may be a very pleasant experience, but the kind used is rather different from that which you would normally get in the West. It should be called acupressure, although there are three other types of massage like this which use almost identical points. These other techniques are referred to as Shiatsu, Kiatsu, and G-Jo. The technique involves using firm pressing or circular movements on the specific points. The principle is again rather like rubbing a tender part to relieve a pain, but with the added idea that it is possible to redistribute the flow of energy in the body. This form of massage forms the basis for a most useful technique for dealing with established headaches, or even preventing their occurrence. You can either use the technique on yourself, or else have somebody else do it for you.

There are four points on each side of the head and neck which typically become tender before a headache develops. As the headache progresses these points become more and more tender. If these are injected with a local anaesthetic it is often possible to terminate a headache. It has also proven possible to stop the majority of attacks either by gently pushing a fine needle into these points, or else by simply applying a firm circular pressure for ten minutes or so.

These four points are to be found in the following places:

1 On the upper border of the muscle running from the neck to the shoulder, halfway between the shoulder tip and the neck;
2 At the back of the skull, at each end of the place where the muscle is attached;
3 In the middle of the temple, if you feel gently, you will find a small depression, and this is the correct point;
4 Just above the root of the nose, at the tips of the eyebrows.

If you press on each of these points you will find them easily. They may be slightly tender if you press on them. In the hours before an attack of headache develops, and particularly if it is migraine, all these points become more tender, but especially the ones on the side where the headache will eventually be. If, immediately you notice the tenderness, you begin firm, circular pressure on each of these points in turn, you have a good chance of aborting the headache. It is as well to apply the pressure to all the eight points and not just the most tender ones, otherwise the headache may just develop somewhere else. It is very important always to do it on both sides. The normal recommendation is to do about two minutes on each point. It is very uncommon for all this pressure actually to cause a headache, but if it does, then this technique is not for you.

Acupuncture and acupressure are undoubtedly effective forms of treatment, but it is important to go to a fully trained and registered practitioner, and with the full knowledge of your doctor. As with the majority of the alternative therapies, acupuncture in most Western countries has now organised itself and keeps registers of people who have undergone a minimum training. If you want to try this form of treatment, then either ask your doctor if he will recommend someone or else find out if the therapist is on the register. You can then reassure yourself that he or she will be both adequately trained and likely to behave ethically. There are some details of registers in the back of the book.

We have given a broad outline of how the acupuncturist thinks his treatments work, although this explanation is impossible to understand in terms of conventional medical science. If we assume that acupuncture does something more than just administer a hefty placebo, is there a possibility of some scientific explanation? Well, perhaps there is. It does appear to alter the balance of various chemicals in the brain, and this alteration may provide a rationale for its effect in headache.

CHAPTER SIX

Homoeopathic Treatments

Throughout the world, the use of homoeopathic medicine is growing very rapidly, and this growth has been particularly marked in the West. It is practised both by doctors and lay practitioners, and homoeopathic remedies are freely available for use by the public. In Britain, homoeopathic treatment has for many years been available under the National Health Service, and today there are many doctors both in general practice and in the special homoeopathic hospitals who use it in conjunction with conventional treatments.

The basic ideas of homoeopathy have an ancient history. Many of its principles were drawn up and used by the traditional fathers of conventional medicine. For centuries these principles were lost and neglected but in the last 150 years they have gradually re-emerged. The modern founder was Dr Samuel Hahnemann in the early part of the nineteenth century.

Homoeopathic treatment is based on the use of the so-called 'Similar principle', which has also been described as 'Like cures like'. An illness or disease is treated with a remedy which may itself cause similar symptoms. We must explain this in some detail because this idea is central to understanding what happens when you go to see a homoeopathic practitioner. Until recently, many people had to be vaccinated against smallpox. This vaccination is done using a virus which, when active, causes symptoms like mild smallpox. So, using something which causes symptoms like smallpox is used to prevent smallpox itself. We now know it works by stimulating a particular response in the body's immune system. The way in which the smallpox vaccination is used is very much like the basic principle of homoeopathy. Something which causes symptoms like smallpox is used to prevent smallpox itself. The trick was to get the vaccination virus into a form in which it protected the body without doing it harm. Now, homoeopathic remedies are not viruses and do not cause an immune response, but the principle remains the same. Let us take an example.

Jack was a 38-year-old red-haired lorry driver, with a bright red face and fat waist, who had been suffering with severe headaches for the last ten years. These were typical tension headaches which occurred after driving for long periods. He had in the past had a number of episodes of migraine, some attacks being of the classical type with flashing lights in front of the eyes, but most being common migraine. He had tried a lot of different treatments but was now becoming worried that the headaches were going to interfere with his job. He came from an area of high unemployment and the prospect of job problems was particularly daunting. He was happily married with four children. He drank eight or nine pints of beer each weekend and smoked forty cigarettes each day. His general practitioner had recently taken on a new junior partner who had taken some postgraduate courses in homoeopathy, and it was suggested that Jack might like to be treated using this method. He was rather sceptical but the urgency of his situation convinced him that it was worth trying some new approach. The new doctor took a very full history from Jack. He admitted that he was generally a rather lively person but was sometimes given to having violent tempers, particularly when he had a headache. When he had a headache his normally red face would shine like a beetroot and he would feel that his whole face and head were throbbing. He often had a dry hacking cough which he thought was due to his heavy smoking. Although he had thought that his headaches occurred primarily after driving, it soon became clear that the headaches in fact tended to occur in the afternoons and at night, and were made much worse by noise. The doctor prescribed a homoeopathic preparation of Belladonna, and Jack's headaches became gradually much better over the next four weeks. He has remained headache free since then, and further homoeopathic treatments have been used to help him to stop smoking.

The homoeopath goes into the details of the complaint rather more comprehensively than other practitioners would. While taking the normal medical history, he or she is particularly concerned with other, general, symptoms which conventional medical practitioners would probably not link with your headaches. He will be interested to know, for example, how you react to cold or heat or extremes of these. Most of us tend to favour one type of temperature or weather, but in some people, especially when they are ill, this becomes accentuated. They may feel generally run down and lifeless when it is hot, but their headaches improve. It is these odd symptoms which are crucial to the homoeopath. There are other important features which he will ask about: have you noticed if you feel better in the open air or indoors? Do you perspire a lot? Are there any particular times of the day when you get headaches? How do you sleep, and do you ever remember any of your dreams? Strong food likes or dislikes, if they are not influenced by advice, habit or religion may well be relevant. The answers to all of these may be very helpful in deciding on the remedy. The factors which modify symptoms are known as 'modalities'.

From all this information he will build up a total picture of you, constructed of two closely linked parts. One part is your 'constitutional type'. This is similar to what psychologists refer to as your personality 'traits' — those life-long emotional predispositions to things. The other part is how you are reacting to your current situation, which is largely dependent on your headaches. It is this which varies all the time during your life and will continue to change as treatment proceeds. It roughly corresponds to what psychologists call your personality 'state'.

The onset of the illness, even if this occurred many years earlier, is another point which the homoeopath will go into in some detail. Did the headaches first start after the loss of someone close to you, or after some profound emotional experience or anger, or is there something to suggest a long-standing resentment about something which has happened in your life? Did they perhaps start after a fall or after a fright. Things which the conventional doctor would probably consider to be of minor importance. These questions are not just asked because of their psychological implications but also because they may point towards specific remedies. There will also be questions about family history, in particular whether there are any diseases which run in the family. Although the history is of prime importance to the homoeopath, do not worry if you cannot answer all the questions. All medical practitioners, whether conventional or homoeopathic, know how difficult it is to remember everything in detail.

During all this extensive history-taking, the homoeopathic physician will be observing you closely, and these observations supply one more important ingredient before he can proceed to the next stage. This involves consulting a book known as a 'repertory'. There are several of these in common use, and in essence they are all collections of many thousands of symptoms. By cross-checking your symptoms against those in the book he arrives at the appropriate remedy. It is remarkable that this process of matching your symptoms with those of certain remedies, which takes only a few minutes, will almost invariably point to just one remedy from the 2,000 or so which are listed. Some homoeopaths now use a small computer to help them find the correct remedy, and more will probably do so in the future. However, there are occasions when the history is so clear cut that it is not necessary to go to the repertory. Jack was just one of these extremely clear-cut cases. Let us see why.

In any of the standard books on homoeopathy, the people who need Belladonna are described as red-faced, plethoric, and fat. They tend to be lively, entertaining people when they are well, but when they become ill, they become bad-tempered and even violent. Interestingly, the men tend more often to be red haired. When they are ill, they become very red faced, and the whole head feels hot and painful. At the same time, the mouth may go dry, and be associated with a dry, hacking cough. So much for the main features of the headache which could fit for very many different homoeopathic remedies, but it was the modifying features of the headaches — the modalities — which narrowed down the search for the right remedy. The headaches associated with Belladonna are aggravated by noise, touch and motion, and they typically become worse after 3 o'clock in the afternoon and at night. They may also be brought on or worsened by drinking and by lying down, but be relieved by rest. So the history, and Jack's general appearance, fitted very well with the description of Belladonna and this was the only remedy which would really have been of use.

The next question, is how have these lists of symptoms been assembled? They are based upon one of the other things peculiar to homoeopathy. These are the 'provings'. It was Hahnemann who first noticed that the toxic symptoms of a particular drug sometimes exactly corresponded to the symptoms of certain diseases. He then hit upon the idea of using a dilute solution of the toxic compound to treat the disease. He matched the symptoms produced by the drug in overdosage with the symptoms of the disease to decide which drug to use for which disease. Again, the idea of like curing like. Homoeopaths since Hahnemann's time have used information on poisonings, and have also experimented with all sorts of different compounds to discover their effects in normal healthy people. Giving minute doses of a remedy to normal volunteers, and monitoring their reactions, is what is meant by the 'provings'. Over the years, all this information has been put together into the homoeopathic Materia Medica, the grand list of all the remedies used. There are now well over 2,000 different remedies listed, and for many of the remedies there are hundreds of different symptoms listed. Taking all the symptoms and features together makes it possible to build up a picture of the symptoms characteristic of a remedy. The repertory, which we mentioned earlier, is the key to this enormous list of symptoms. It is the selection of a treatment on the basis of a matching of the patient's symptoms with the symptom picture of the remedy which lies at the heart of homoeopathic practice.

Having decided on the appropriate remedy, all that is now left is to decide on the correct dose. Many people are dismayed when they are only given a single dose of the remedy, and then left alone for three or four weeks to see what happens. Many of the potent remedies are in fact best given in this way and there is no advantage in taking more of the remedy. Unlike conventional treatments, taking more of a remedy does not add to the benefit which it may do you. This in itself is sometimes difficult to understand but it is a most important point. There are several possible results of homoeopathic treatment, and it must be stressed that there is little relationship between the severity of the symptoms and your response. You may experience no effect at all, you may transiently become worse, or you may improve. Apart from these fairly obvious alternatives, the homoeopath also looks for variations on these themes, and they will guide his next move.

The second time that he sees you, the homoeopath will again take a brief history in order to establish whether you have had a reaction. At this stage, a reaction does not necessarily mean an improvement, it is your overall response which counts. Homoeopathy aims to deal with the root causes of your headaches and cure will almost invariably take much longer. This is yet another difference from conventional medicine where the aim is to get a rapid cure, but the emphasis is on dealing with headache symptoms rather than underlying causes, which are poorly understood. At this second consultation, the homoeopath will decide if you should have a further dose, or some different remedy. If he sees clear evidence of a good reaction, he may even decide to leave you a while longer without interfering.

Although the remedy that is used will be tailor-made to your requirements, there are a small number of homoeopathic remedies that are used more often than others in the treatment of headache. This is because, as with acupuncture diagnosis, even if ultimately all people are separate individuals, their symptoms do fall into certain categories. These remedies can be bought over the counter and used, without the need for going to a homoeopath. In Britain and the United States, it is the usual practice to take only one remedy at a time, but some practitioners may use remedies in combination. This is a popular way of using them in some parts of continental Europe. It is not clear whether the single remedy idea is important or not and homoeopaths have different views on this.

The remedies are harmless in themselves and if you take the wrong one it will just not work. Side-effects probably never happen except perhaps with the very potent preparations, which you will not be sold unless on prescription. Although the remedies themselves are safe, we must again make the point that one potential hazard about using homoeopathic remedies is that you may continue to take them when in fact you need some other form of treatment. If your headaches have come on suddenly, are severe or are deteriorating, you should not start trying to treat yourself. Go and have a check up from your doctor.

In general, the author is not enthusiastic about people trying to diagnose and treat themselves, but is well aware that this is an increasing trend. It is therefore important that you should have accurate information on what to do. In the case of chronic, or even just of occasional irritating headaches, these homoeo-pathic remedies can be immensely valuable, and the risk of taking them unsupervised is minimal. If you are going to try using these it is best to use either the 6C or the 12C preparations — we explain what these numbers mean later in this section. When you take the remedy, you place it in your mouth and let it slowly dissolve. It is said that you should not smoke or use strong toothpaste for the hour or so before you take the remedy. During a headache you take one tablet every two hours. For more chronic cases you take one three times a day between meals. You stop taking the remedy when the headaches have stopped. Occasionally when taking remedies you may get an aggravation: the symptoms transiently become worse. If this happens, postpone the next doses until this phase has passed. Finally, do not handle the tablets. Tip them into the lid of their container and then drop them into your mouth.

For historical reasons the remedies are typically given Latin names, and listed below are details of a few of those which are used most commonly in headache. If you find that you fit the list of symptoms accompanying one of these remedies, then it may be the one for you to use. It is important to remember that headaches may have many different causes, and if, for instance, they are the result of ear problems then you may need quite a different set of remedies. There are also different remedies to use during the time that you actually have a headache, and for the prevention and treatment of chronic headaches.

For use during a headache

Gelsemium is a remedy normally used for treating the symptoms of influenza, but it can be useful for dealing with some forms of headache, particularly those tight ones occurring at the back of the head, which are worse in damp, mild weather. The symptoms are invariably worse around 10 am, and are often associated with aches in the muscles. The headache tends to be relieved by passing a large amount of urine.

Iris Versicolor is a remedy which has been found to be very useful in acute migraine. The headache associated with this remedy tends to be at the front of the head, or to feel rather constricting. It is usually accompanied by some nausea or vomiting, and the headache tends to come on after mental strain, especially while relaxing — the typical 'weekend headache'. A rather odd feature is that the headache is often made worse by rest, but improved by moving about.

Sanguinaria is often the remedy for headaches occurring on the right side of the head, and recurring primarily before the menstrual period. The headache typically starts in the morning, but gradually improves in the course of the day. It is associated with dizziness and nausea, and is improved by lying down or going to sleep. It often seems to cut short or at least reduce the severity of the headache. It is also sometimes of value in treating the headaches caused by spending too much time in the sun.

Spigelia is a remedy which is associated with pains primarily on the left side of the head. They tend to be shooting pains which extend down to the face and arm, and are worse on moving about or stooping. It is another remedy for headaches occurring before or immediately after the menstrual period.

Glonoine is used for headaches that feel as if they are bursting, with a violent pounding of the head in time with the pulse. These headaches are sometimes brought on by exposure to heat or the sun.

Bryonia is said to be more often helpful to people who have dark hair and complexion. Pains tend to be right-sided, but the important thing is that the symptoms become much worse on movement. Moving either the head or the eyes leads to a dramatic increase in the intensity of the pain, but surprisingly, pressure on the affected part, or lying on the painful side may improve the symptoms. People who require this remedy are usually very dry; they are thirsty, with dry lips, and may even have a dry cough.

China Sulph headaches start as an ache in the back of the head which rapidly spreads over the whole head, which feels sweaty and damp. The headache is made worse by being in the open air and by turning the head or eyes. The person often looks and feels nauseated, but still wants to eat.

For use during chronic headaches or between attacks

The remedy is often not as clear cut as it is during the acute headache attack. The homoeopath will normally take all the features of the person into account. The mental symptoms, as well as the modifying factors must all be considered in trying to find the correct remedy. Many homoeopaths claim considerable success in reducing the frequency and severity of migraine attacks by prescribing in this way.

Kali Bichromicum is a frequently used remedy for the prevention of headaches. Typically the symptoms start at the root of the nose, and are associated with a lot of sticky catarrh or a badly blocked nose. This is often the remedy for people who get headaches from sinus trouble. The pains tend to be worse on moving or on stooping, but are improved by being out in the open air and eating hot things. The patient dislikes the heat and may have a yellowish appearance. The pains tend to occur in small areas rather than all over the head.

Natrum Muriaticum is made from common salt. The symptoms are those of classical migraine, with a hammering type of headache preceded or accompanied by flashing zigzags in front of the eyes, or even a brief partial loss of vision. The eyes tend to water, and the symptoms are all worse between the afternoon and the evening. The headache tends to come and go in fairly regular cycles. People who benefit from this remedy often have rather greasy skins, perhaps with spots, and to be shy and nervous. It is usually recommended that this remedy should be avoided during the acute headache phase.

The remedy *Lachesis* is used especially in menopausal women with a particular type of headache, which is present when they wake up in the morning. The pain is pulsating or hammering, and the face sometimes looks purplish, with puffy eyes. More often than not the symptoms are on the left side and improved by cold weather. The person who needs this may feel jealous and suspicious for no obvious reason.

The headache of *Sepia* is usually associated with nausea, and all the symptoms tend to be improved by having a sleep. It is almost unique in that the headache of the *Sepia* person improves on violent exertion. These folk tend to be irritable and weepy, and although normally tidy, they become indifferent to themselves, their houses and families.

Cimicifuga is said to be a useful remedy in people who have headaches at the back of the head which feel as if they are pressing upwards. People say that they feel that the top of their head will shoot off. There is often also some aching in the muscles of the neck. This is another of the remedies which is used for women who get headaches before their menstrual periods, particularly if they are feeling gloomy. This sort of person tends to be very changeable both in mental and physical symptoms.

Silica headaches usually also start in the back of the head and extend over the top towards the eyes. They tend to occur more often on the right and to have a bursting feeling. The whole head tends to be very sensitive to draughts and noise. Sometimes the headache is associated with a brief loss of vision and even numbness in the arm. These people tend to have clammy feet and hands, to feel chilly, and to have a dread of failure. They become exhausted easily.

This is by no means an exhaustive list of the remedies used in the treatment of headache but the list will enable most people to find a suitable remedy. If you do not recognise yourself in this list, but would like to follow this approach to treatment, then you should go to a homoeopath.

In Britain, if you want to have homoeopathic treatment your general practitioner can refer you, and you can have free treatment under the National Health Service. Alternatively, he may suggest a non-medical homoeopath, and the usual rule applies about finding somebody who is trained and registered. Details about this are in the appendix.

The idea of 'like treating like' is still regarded with considerable scepticism by the medical profession in general, but as we pointed out in our example of smallpox vaccination, the principle is actually used in certain areas of conventional medicine. It is considerably more difficult to understand the homoeopathic idea that the infinitesimally small doses which are used can have a therapeutic effect. The basic substance from which the remedy is made may be of animal, vegetable or mineral origin. The raw material is crushed and an alcoholic extract made by a process of soaking and filtering. Then begins the process of making the diluted homoeopathic remedy. One drop of the alcoholic extract is added to ten or a hundred drops of alcohol or an alcohol and water mixture. It is then vigorously shaken either by hand or by machine. This shaking is called 'succussion', and this is regarded as the important part of making a homoeopathic remedy. The preparation is more than just making dilutions. Some remedies which are insoluble are made using lactose powder as the diluting substance instead. The diluting process is continued for a standard number of times to produce the final remedy which can be prescribed or bought. In practice, there are certain standard dilutions which are used. Most often these are the so-called 6C, 12C or 30C preparations and can be bought over the counter in many pharmacies, and even in some health food shops. The 'C' means that the remedy has been diluted a hundredfold at each stage in its preparation. The number indicates how many times this dilution has been carried out. With the 12C preparation, the dilution of one drop in a hundred drops has been carried out twelve times. Simple arithmetic reveals that the final product has been diluted to such an extent that one part of the original now exists in

1,000,000,000,000 parts of the solution. The 12C and 30C preparations do not actually contain any of the original substance, and the problem for the medical scientist is the idea that something which contains just alcohol and water can have any kind of effect on either the body or the mind. Other even more dilute remedies designated 1M and 10M are often prescribed and, according to homoeopaths, these are even more potent. It does seem that this principle of increasing potency with increasing dilution is contrary to common sense. But many ideas that have at first seemed illogical have ultimately been shown to have some truth in them. Rather than worrying about the logic of the idea it is more sensible to have a look at the evidence. At the moment there is not much apart from simple uncontrolled observations, but it will be important for all of us to keep an open mind in the future if we are to avoid losing potentially valuable treatments.

Anecdotes about the effectiveness of homoeopathy do not cut much ice with the sceptic. So, is there any scientific evidence that homoeopathic treatment actually works? There have been many attempts to show that the potentised remedies have effects in the laboratory, some of which do seem to demonstrate that there is an effect which cannot be explained using our normal scientific model. All these experiments are being repeated at the moment, and so we must wait to see what these scientists discover. Others have been performing a number of clinical trials on homoeopathic remedies, and it does look as if some remedies do have a significant effect which cannot be explained away on the basis of a placebo response. There have not yet been any trials of homoeopathy in headache, and so we cannot give a scientific answer to the question, does it work? All we can say at this stage is that extensive observations lead us to think that homoeopathic treatment may be very valuable for some people.

CHAPTER SEVEN

Hypnosis

It is only in recent years that hypnosis has come to be seen as a relatively respectable form of treatment. For many years it was regarded with great hostility, and in many countries its practice was severely restricted by various laws. It has now largely come in from the cold and is used for a wide range of illnesses, emotional and psychological conditions and personality problems. It is primarily practised by doctors or dentists who have had special training, or by clinical psychologists who are usually attached to hospital psychiatric departments. In most Western countries there are also a number of lay hypnotherapists in practice, but unfortunately the quality and quantity of their training is very variable.

Hypnosis has a fascinating past. It has been used in some form or other throughout history, and although outside the scope of this book, the interested reader may pursue the references at the back. There is now a wealth of scientific data to prove its effectiveness in a large number of clinical situations, including headache.

Until quite recently, hypnosis had a very bad image. There were highly inaccurate representations of it in films and the media, and many still associate it with something vaguely sinister. There may be those who have used hypnosis to affect individuals adversely, but it must be emphasised that therapeutic hypnosis cannot be administered against your will; you remain in control of yourself throughout the hypnotic session. It is essentially a method for enabling you to use the powers of your own mind but there is nothing mystical about it. The hypnotist does not require any special personality traits, and indeed it is a technique that can be successfully learnt by most people. Similarly, although some people are better hypnotic subjects than others, it is rare to find someone who genuinely cannot be hypnotised. It is important to stress that there is no connection between the ease with which someone can be hypnotised and either their intelligence or gullibility.

In recent years, there has been a lot of discussion about whether the hypnotic state even exists. Many of us routinely enter states just like mild hypnosis, for instance if we are watching a film, or even just looking at the scenery from a car or train. So perhaps being hypnotised represents no more than a variation on a common state of consciousness. This is an important theoretical issue, but since we are concerned here more with the practicalities of hypnosis, we shall use a simple model to try to explain what happens during therapeutic hypnosis. In many respects, the hypnotic state is rather like the earliest stage of sleep. It is a very relaxing experience during which some of the normal critical faculties of the mind are partially suspended. It therefore becomes possible for the hypnotherapist to communicate with your subconscious mind. We normally all have a number of barriers which may prevent contact with the deeper parts of ourselves. It is these barriers which we can sometimes get round by using hypnosis.

Jean was a 54-year-old housewife who worked part-time in a local supermarket. She had suffered with migraine for many years, but the attacks had gradually stopped at the time of the menopause. She was now having regular episodes of generalised tension headaches. These were occurring every day and were severely interfering with her life. They became worse on the days when she worked in the supermarket, and recently she had started waking with these headaches. She was becoming very worried about them, fearing that there might be something seriously wrong with her. Her worries were almost certainly making the headaches worse. She had been on a number of different treatments, including pain killers, anti-depressants and tranquillisers. Her doctor re-examined her to reassure her that there was nothing sinister causing her symptoms. Jean felt that she did not want to continue taking medications if they were not helping her, and asked whether there was any other form of treatment that she could try. Her doctor arranged for her to see another doctor who practised hypnotherapy. She was given a total of three sessions, during which she was taught how to deal with some of the situations which were triggering the headaches, and how to use a simple technique for reducing the headaches when they did occur. She was considerably improved, and this improvement has been maintained for over a year. She only rarely takes any pain killers and is not on any regular medications.

If it is decided to treat you with hypnosis, it will probably take place in the normal consulting room. You will first be made comfortable, usually sitting in a chair. Sometimes you will be asked to lie on a couch, just because this can be still more comfortable and help you to relax. It is helpful if the room is kept at an agreeable temperature and the lighting dimmed.

It will be important for the hypnotherapist to establish that you really want to have this form of treatment, and he or she will usually ask a few specific questions about you and your feelings towards hypnosis, and in particular if you have any fears or apprehensions about it. As we said, this form of hypnosis will not and cannot be administered against your will, and it is essential to ensure that you do not have any resistance to the idea of being hypnotised. For this reason he or she will also be interested in your previous knowledge of hypnosis, and will try to find out if you have any misconceptions about it. Most hypnotherapists will offer an explanation about what they will do, and what will happen. This discussion phase is essential in order to ensure that you are in the right state of mind to fully participate in the session. As with every other form of treatment, success depends upon your willingness to help the therapist to help you. No treatment can ever be fully effective if you expect someone to do something to you, rather than doing it together. This is especially true of hypnotherapy.

After the discussions, the next part of hypnosis is known as 'induction'. It is the actual process of helping you to get into the hypnotic state. Note that it is to help you to get there, not forcing you into something. There are many ways of inducing hypnosis but the most commonly used is to start with eye fixation. You are asked to stare at some object while the hypnotherapist gradually starts to talk to you. He or she will then suggest that you close your eyes and just follow the various suggestions which are made to you. The hypnotherapist will commonly use some simple exercises, to slow and regularise your breathing. At this point you will almost certainly be in a mild hypnotic state. It really is as simple as that. People report all sorts of different experiences while hypnotised. Many say that they felt that they could have just opened their eyes at any time and terminated the session. This does not mean that they were not hypnotised, but it does show once again that the hypnotic state is largely voluntary.

The first advantage of being in the hypnotic state is that it is possible to become very relaxed. It is then easy to respond to more and more of the suggestions which the hypnotherapist presents to you, and you will probably feel that you want to. The main thrust of what you do now with the hypnotherapist depends on the exact nature of the problem. For instance, if you have found that you normally get headaches in response to stressful situations, you may start to work on ways of responding differently to stress. Alternatively, he or she may help you to see if there are some psychological causes for the headaches and to deal with them. The remarkable thing is that suggestions made and work done, during hypnosis, actually have an effect on you after the session is over.

At the end of the hypnotic session, you are gradually returned to normal consciousness. There is some skill in doing this well, so that you do not lose any of the positive things gained during the session. If you terminate the session too rapidly, as sometimes happens if people stop it themselves, then it is possible to lose everything that you have gained. The only areas of life which will be affected by the hypnosis will be those specifically dealt with during the session. You will not be left with any sort of unwanted effects. You might be left with so-called post hypnotic suggestions. For instance, if during the session you dealt with the way that you get headaches whenever anybody at work tells you off, you may have been left with a suggestion that you would automatically start to relax if this occurs. Finally, some hypnotherapists make a lot of use of autohypnosis. While hypnotised they teach you how to achieve the same state while you are on your own. This approach can be very valuable for people who suffer from headaches in response to specific happenings in their lives.

Although hypnosis is becoming widely used in conventional medical practice, it has proved difficult to investigate it in the accepted scientific way. Largely because hypnosis seems to be a very common occurrence in daily life, it is difficult to define it accurately. Over the years there have been a number of attempts to define accurately the various levels of hypnosis. It is difficult to do this, and now most scientific work defines hypnosis in terms of scales of susceptibility; the most susceptible people will enter a hypnotic state easily, and without an involved induction procedure, while the least susceptible need considerable preparation to enter even the earliest stages. It is becoming clear that the psychology of hypnosis is a complicated subject, and although a lengthy discussion of it is not possible here, the references at the back will provide more information. However, what is clear is that it is possible to use hypnosis for the effective treatment of a wide range of different conditions, and that headache is an important one of these.

CHAPTER EIGHT

Biofeedback and Relaxation

Although we are including biofeedback and relaxation in the section on alternative approaches to treatment, both are now widely used by conventional headache specialists, and both are of proven value in the treatment of all forms of headache.

During the 1960s, biofeedback was the fashionable form of treatment for all sorts of different illnesses, and there were claims that it could be used for inducing a variety of desirable states of consciousness. In the intervening years there has been a lot of careful research which has shown that there are a small number of illnesses in which the technique may be beneficial. One of these is headache.

Biofeedback is essentially a method of teaching people to become aware of the functioning of various parts of their own bodies. Once they have been taught this, they are then trained to alter the activity of whichever part is causing trouble. This may sound complicated, but in practice it is very simple. In headache, two different types of biofeedback are used.

The first is electrical biofeedback, in which the patient is attached to a machine which records electrical activity in the muscles around the scalp. The machine represents the amount of activity in the muscles by means of a flashing light or a sound. We know that people with chronic headaches have a lot of activity in these muscles, and so at the beginning of the session there are a lot of sounds or flashing lights. You are then asked to reduce the sounds or the lights. As the muscles become more relaxed, the lights or sounds do indeed start to reduce in intensity. With subsequent sessions the reduction in intensity continues, together with an increase in the relaxation of the muscles. Most people are able to use this technique, and in a proportion of patients the frequency and severity of the headaches are markedly reduced.

The second type of biofeedback is based upon temperature control. Small heat sensitive monitors are put either on the scalp or on the hands, and again the patient is trained to control the temperature of the monitored part. This may seem a little far-fetched, but experiments have shown that after only an hour's training virtually anyone can learn to raise the temperature of one hand by one or two degrees Centigrade. This means that the patient can then learn to control the flow of blood around the scalp, which is supposed to be of importance in headache. The technique may, in fact, work by teaching the patient how to relax.

Helen was a dark haired 37-year-old administrator in the communications industry. She had a very busy and stressful job which involved a great deal of travelling. She had been having serious tension headaches for the last five years which were gradually becoming worse. During her middle 20s she had suffered with common migraine during the time that she was taking the oral contraceptive pill. The attacks of migraine had ceased within three months of stopping it, and she had then had no further problems until the tension headaches started. In her attempts to rid herself of these headaches she had tried a variety of dietary manoeuvres and had stopped smoking, but nothing seemed to help. Her doctor treated her successfully with a mild sedative and some pain killers, but she became very worried that these drugs might interfere with her ability to do her job. She asked to see another doctor and was subsequently treated with electrical biofeedback. The results were rapid and gratifying. She was able to attend for a total of six treatments over a period of three months and there was a major reduction in the frequency and severity of the headaches.

In general, electrical biofeedback is used more often for

tension headache, and temperature biofeedback for migraine, although there are exceptions to this rule. We are not yet able to predict which patients will respond to this technique, and who will not. In the past, one difficulty was that patients tended to be referred for biofeedback only after everything else had failed, and such people tend to be notoriously difficult to treat. The equipment required is still only available in special centres but hopefully it will become more widely available in the future.

The main benefit of biofeedback appears to be that it induces a state of controlled relaxation. It is possible for most people to learn relaxation techniques without the use of any special equipment, but it does require a little more effort. We know that tension is an important factor in all headaches, not just the sensation of feeling tense but tension in muscles as well. The use of a relaxation technique of some sort will help many, if not most headache sufferers, and it is worth learning one, whatever form of treatment you decide to go for.

There are a number of sophisticated techniques for making you feel more relaxed and less tense — things like Yoga, autogenic training and T'ai Chi Ch'uan. The initial aim of the sort of relaxation training which we are discussing is not to make you more calm and relaxed, but to alter the way in which your body deals with tension. As time goes by you do indeed become more relaxed but that is not the first aim. Almost anyone can learn a simple relaxation technique — the author has seen a small boy under 10 as well as a lady in her 80s learn successfully. Very occasionally, people who are extremely tense develop more headaches as they begin to use the method, and this appears to be a reaction of the body to the new situation of being relaxed. It is worth persisting, but if the headaches continue to become worse then it is best to stop and seek the advice of your doctor.

Relaxation techniques usually need 10 to 15 minutes twice a day, and most people can learn the technique in six to eight weeks. With practice, the time needed to perform the exercises is markedly reduced, and the benefit spreads throughout the day. It is most important to continue with the exercises even when the headaches have gone, to reduce the chance of them recurring. Before starting the exercises, it is a good idea to try to increase the amount of physical exercise you take each day, to help improve your general condition. It is also valuable to get into the habit of spending as little time as possible fixed in one position; for example, a secretary should stop typing for a minute or two every hour, and sit up straight and have a stretch. Chronic bad posture is probably the cause of some headaches. At the same time, try to eat regular balanced meals, and to reduce the amount of red meat which you eat. Smokers should not smoke immediately before or after the exercises. Relaxation techniques can often be very helpful to people who want to stop smoking.

There are two commonly used exercises which can be recommended:

1   Lie flat on your back on the floor, with a small pillow or two or three books under the back of the head — the idea is to keep the neck and spine straight during the exercise. Your knees should then be drawn up so that they are comfortably bent. If necessary you can use a pillow to support them. Close your eyes and take slow regular breaths in and out through your nose. Do not hold your breath. Continue with this slow, regular breathing for 3 or 4 minutes. This will be relaxing in itself. Then start to make a conscious effort to relax your muscles. Start at your feet and gradually work up the body until you finish with your head and neck. Some people find it useful to tense the muscles first before allowing them to become completely heavy and relaxed. Before long you will feel those areas in your muscles that remain stubbornly tense and you will need to put a little extra effort into these. Carry on for a total of about 15 minutes and then gradually straighten your legs and sit up slowly.

2   Sit upright in a chair, preferably one with a firm back, with your feet flat on the floor in a comfortable position. Sit in a relaxed upright posture, ensuring that your neck and spine are straight, but without straining, and with your hands resting in your lap. As in the previous exercise, close your eyes and start regular, slow, comfortable breathing through your nose. Continue doing this for 3 or 4 minutes and then concentrate on relaxing your muscles, starting at the feet and working your way up the body. The whole exercise should be done for about 15 minutes.

This exercise is particularly valuable because, once mastered, you can use the same technique while sitting at a desk or typewriter. Relaxation can be induced very rapidly even under those situations.

As you get better at using these techniques, the benefit lasts progressively longer and it becomes easier and easier to relax yourself. Many people have successfully learnt to relax themselves out of a headache just as it is developing.

It is sometimes necessary to introduce other relaxation exercises which may need to be tailored to your particular requirements.

Some people have found great benefit from practising Yoga, particularly if they have found an experienced teacher who is used to dealing with minor physical problems like excess tension in muscles. Yoga is a very ancient system. Most people associate it with sequences of contorted postures, the so-called Hatha Yoga. For the serious practitioner, this type is actually only used to prepare and organise the body and the mind for some of the more advanced types of Yoga. There are dozens of different schools of Yoga and they all consider spiritual enlightenment as their ultimate goal. In recent years, there has been a lot of research into the physical and emotional effects of Yoga, and some use specific postures and breathing techniques for treatment. There is some evidence that Yoga can benefit people with headaches. However, it must be used with caution; some postures, especially the inverted ones, may make headaches worse if they are used indiscriminately. Yoga has a great deal to offer in many different illnesses, and the best way to ensure that you benefit is to get a competent, trained teacher. If you want to take up Yoga, go and see the teacher first and tell him or her that you have headaches, and what they are like. The teacher can then select specific exercises for you to do and warn you about any which may cause you problems.

CHAPTER NINE

Manipulating the Body

Osteopathy, chiropractice and Alexander therapy

Many headaches are the result of problems in the neck and spine. Conventional medicine has only in recent years started to try to tackle the problem of headaches caused in this way, and treatment is still most unsatisfactory. There exists a number of alternative methods of dealing with these problems, the most widely known being osteopathy, chiropractice and Alexander therapy. There are a number of important differences between them, although there are general similarities which lead us to consider them together. The author has seen all three successfully treat headaches which had failed to respond to any other method of treatment.

Osteopathy and *chiropractice* are two similar systems of treatment which have been shown to be of great benefit for dealing with problems associated with bones, joints and ligaments. Problems at these sites may cause nerves to be trapped and chiropractice in particular attempts to relieve trapped or squashed nerves. There are differences in philosophy and approach in these two systems but for our purposes they can be considered together. Each works on the spine, although the osteopath regularly works on other parts of the body as well.

There are now stringent training requirements for anyone wishing to become a registered osteopath or chiropractor, and the ruling bodies insist on the highest standards of professional conduct. In some parts of the world, certain chiropractors have made extravagant claims concerning some of the things they can treat, and this has led to all chiropractors being viewed with a certain amount of scepticism in these countries. This is a great shame because most do have a great deal to offer the patient suffering from headache who has not responded to other forms of treatment. They seem to have the most to offer people who have headaches as a result of pains in the neck or a history of back trouble, as well as headaches, or in those in whom the headaches started after some accident or injury. As with all forms of therapy, they cannot treat all headaches, but if you and your doctor feel that you fall into one of these categories and the approach appeals to you, then they may be worth considering.

Patricia was a 41-year-old secretary who had been suffering from chronic headaches for almost twenty years. Some attacks were undoubtedly migrainous but others were more like tension headaches. She had tried an enormous range of different pain killers and tranquillisers over the years but none had been particularly successful. She then woke one day with a severe attack of low back pain. She visited her general practitioner several times and after the failure of all the usual forms of treatment, he suggested that she should consult a local osteopath. She went to see the osteopath, who was promptly able to deal with her back pain. He followed this with some general advice on how to strengthen her back and to change to a much firmer mattress. He then set about trying to treat her headaches. It was the osteopath's feeling that the headaches were being caused by problems in the neck and he treated her neck a total of four times. At the end of this, her headaches had almost vanished and she has remained largely headache free since that time.

There is one other type of osteopathy which seems particularly improbable to those who are medically trained — this is cranial osteopathy, where all the manipulations are done on the head. It is claimed that the bones of the head are moved but this seems unlikely, since the skull bones cease to be mobile after early childhood. Since the technique does appear to help some patients, it is either working via our old friend the placebo response, or else it may be having some other action which none of us yet fully understands.

The *Alexander principle* is in some ways similar to the fundamental ideas of the chiropractic and osteopathic schools. It is in essence a method of re-education of posture rather than a therapy as such. The Alexander practitioner considers that many ills, including headaches, are caused by the chronic maintenance of bad posture. It is said that bad posture causes the normal reflexes of the body to be inhibited; for instance, you do not move as smoothly and as effortlessly as you could. This does seem to be an important method with far-reaching consequences, but we have so far only seen it used to prevent the development of further episodes of headache rather than treating an already established case.

Reflexology

Reflexology is an ancient technique in which the soles of the feet are massaged deeply. The technique probably originated in India and China and was largely unknown in the West until the early part of this century.

The practitioner of reflexology considers that there is a flow of energy in the body, a similar idea to that which guides traditional Chinese medicine. The various organs of the body are thought to be represented by certain areas on the sole of the foot. Compressing and massaging these points redirects the flow of energy in the corresponding organ and leads to a cure. For instance, if you have migraine, it might be thought to be due to a disturbance in the flow of energy to the solar plexus. The area on the foot which corresponds to the solar plexus is on the big toe, so this would be one of the first parts of the foot to be massaged.

The reflexologist considers that the circulation of energy in the feet may become sluggish as a result of illness, wearing shoes, or lack of exercise. This is thought to lead to the formation of crystalline deposits, and it is these which can be broken up by massaging the feet. If these deposits are broken down successfully, then the energy can flow again. The correct points to use in different illnesses have been worked out by careful observation over a very long period of time. There are now sophisticated maps showing the location of all the organs of the body on the foot, and there are instructions on how to treat each particular point.

Reflexology has been used by only a few patients known to the author, but the results have been interesting in all of them. None was actually cured, but those with chronic tension headaches reported a remarkable improvement for a matter of some weeks. The treatment is said to be very pleasant. Because the bottoms of the feet are so sensitive, much of the skill of the reflexologist lies in being able to judge the correct amount of pressure to use. You would expect that a gentle massage of your feet might make you feel better, and it is at the present time impossible to say whether the treatments do anything more than this.

CHAPTER TEN

The Causes of Headache: The Research Findings

After many years of relative neglect, headache is at last starting to attract the attention of the scientific and medical communities. There were so many really pressing health problems in the world that many felt that headache was not really worthy of their attention. There have been a few distinguished people over the years who have continued to work in the field, but for the most part it was regarded as little more than a sort of a luxury; headache, it was said, never killed anyone, so why bother to invest scant resources in investigating it. Fortunately, this attitude has been changing in the last few years and there have been some excellent pieces of research performed. Regrettably, much crucial research is still hindered by a lack of funding.

In order to understand something about headache, it is first necessary to think about the phenomenon of pain in general. Probably everybody in the world has suffered a pain at some time in their lives, but there is still a great deal which is not understood about it. For instance, how much of a pain comes from nerves and how much of it starts in the mind itself. There are some people who suffer severe and excruciating pains, even when there is nothing in their bodies causing them. These pains are just as real to them as the pain which someone else might get from a broken leg. The scientific literature on pain is enormous and complicated, but there are a few general themes which have emerged in the last five years or so which have brought some order to the apparent chaos.

Let us consider a pain which actually starts somewhere in the body (we shall leave aside those pains that start in the mind itself). Pain begins when a certain type of nerve fibre is stimulated. If the cause of a pain is sufficiently severe, then every single type of nerve can transmit the sensation. Every other feeling and sensation is blocked out. The nerves carrying information about pain enter the spinal cord and the information is transferred from one nerve to another, until it finally reaches the brain. When it arrives here, you finally experience it. Up to this point, the pain has been something going on outside consciousness. The nerves have been responding to the painful stimulus but you have not known anything about it. On the way to the brain, the painful impulses have to pass through an area known as the brainstem, which lies between the top of the neck and the base of the brain itself. The brainstem contains some of the most remarkable systems in the whole of nature. Everyone has a brainstem, and it is the part of the brain responsible for things like breathing and blood pressure control. It has dozens of separate functions, but the one which concerns us is that it contains a system which is responsible for deciding what sort of nervous impulses reach the brain.

The brainstem is responsible for the 'cocktail party phenomenon'; if you are at a noisy party, it is sometimes difficult to hear what people are saying to you but if you get into conversation with somebody who interests you, you start to focus on what they are saying, and your brain excludes a lot of the surrounding noise. Some people's brains are better at doing this than others. This part of the brain is responsible then for deciding which things from the outside world are going to be allowed to get through to your conscious mind. Very recent research indicates that in the brainstem there is a kind of gate, which only allows pain signals to get through when it is open. When it is closed no pain impulses can get to the brain. We have all heard of soldiers who have not noticed their wounds in the heat of battle. One of the reasons for this is that the brainstem has decided that the time is not right to feel pain. In the same way, some people who have done all the right things to get a headache do not experience it until the 'heat is taken off them', their brainstem decides that they just cannot have a headache at this crucial time, but they certainly will suffer later.

In the brainstem, painful impulses are controlled by a series of specialised nerves. All nerves work by releasing chemicals, and the ones involved most intimately in the control of pain are the endorphins, and a compound known as serotonin or 5-hydroxytryptamine (we met the endorphins in connection with the placebo response, during which they may be released). By damping down the flow of nervous impulses in the brainstem, they can stop you feeling pain. They do have a number of other actions, but their effect on pain is the one in which we are interested here. These endorphins were first isolated during the mid-1970s and the research generated tremendous interest. It was discovered that endorphins have all the effects of the derivatives of opium, but they occur naturally in the brain. Serotonin has many actions throughout the body but its role in pain appears to be particularly crucial in headache.

If you think about it, the only reason for having pain at all is to warn your body that something is going wrong; it is there to tell you if you have put your hand on a fire, or if you have eaten something bad which then gives you a stomach ache. The brainstem should work in such a way that the only things which cause you to feel pain are the things which are liable to damage your body. In headache, it seems that the primary problem is the way in which the brainstem lets painful information get through to the brain. It has been discovered that headache sufferers have a lowered pain threshold all the time, and not just when they have a headache. In a series of experiments designed to measure their appreciation of pain, it was discovered that regular headache sufferers found sounds uncomfortable, and then painful, much sooner than people who never had headaches. Every migraine sufferer will tell you that during the attack, all lights seem brighter and sounds appear louder than they are in reality. This happens to a minor extent whenever we have a pain, but it is never anything like as marked as it is during an attack of headache, and in particular during migraine.

There have been some very careful studies performed recently which have looked into the question of chronic pain. If you have persistent headache for a number of years, then it inevitably starts to change your behaviour. The strongest reaction to severe chronic headache has been shown to be the development of what are known as avoidance behaviours. People begin to avoid certain situations in life. The commonest of these is an avoidance of all social activities and social interactions. The next commonest is the avoidance of household activity, and then of daily travel and movement. As chronic headache persists, depression becomes an important problem. This avoidance behaviour is very common in migraine sufferers, and it is less likely to occur in people with chronic tension headache. Part of the explanation for this appears to be that migraine patients experience more severe pain than do tension headache sufferers, but it is also now very clear that eventually the avoidance behaviours gradually develop a life of their own, making the headache sufferer increasingly sensitive to stimulation in the environment. For instance, as pointed out above, it has been shown that chronic headache sufferers become very sensitive to noise. It is now very clear that successful treatment of chronic pain needs careful attention to these two aspects of the problem — depression and social avoidance, because between them they gradually cause more and more of a feeling of helplessness in the face of the persistent pain.

For many years it was thought that migrainous headaches were due to changes in the behaviour of blood vessels in the scalp and around the brain. It was said that an aura, like flashing lights or numbness down part of one side, that some people experience before migrainous headaches was due to a narrowing of blood vessels around the brain. If a blood vessel narrows, chemical changes occur in the tissues around it and these cause the blood vessel to dilate. It was said that this dilation of the blood vessels of the brain and scalp caused the headache of migraine, in other words, the pain was supposed to be the result of dilated, pulsating blood vessels. This was a persuasive argument and is still accepted by many people. The standard medical textbooks all explain migraine attacks in these terms. Unfortunately, this theory is almost certainly wrong. If you exercise hard, or even if you get into a hot bath, the blood vessels around your head will dilate but you are very unlikely to get a migraine attack. The theory always seemed to make good sense and appeared to be supported by some experiments performed over forty years ago, although it now seems that interpretation of these experiments was faulty. Even during the 1970s further experiments appeared to support this idea of narrowed and then dilated blood vessels. It was maintained that those with common migraine, who do not have an aura, had a generalised narrowing of the blood vessels of the whole of the brain, and that they then developed the painful, dilated pulsating blood vessels. However, an elegant series of experiments from Copenhagen has shown that the old interpretations are untenable, and that the pattern of changes in blood flow around the brain does not happen in the way that had been thought for so many years. Instead, the aura of migraine appears to be caused by a strange phenomenon called 'spreading cortical depression'. In this a slow wave spreads over the surface of the brain itself, damping down and depressing the brain's activity as it goes. As with all new ideas, this one has sparked considerable controversy and we will undoubtedly hear more about it in the years to come.

Blood vessels do undoubtedly have something to do with migraine. During the attack the headache often pounds in time with the pulse. The reason for this seems to be that the brain becomes very sensitive to all sorts of things going on around the head, including the throbbing of blood vessels, whereas normally such pulsing goes unnoticed. This is not the whole explanation. In the same area as the pain gate are the parts of the brainstem which are involved in the control of blood flow in and around the brain. One of the chemicals involved in blood flow around the brain is serotonin. Precisely the same chemical involved in pain control.

It now appears very likely that migraine is caused by a chemical disturbance in the brainstem. This chemical imbalance leads to a change in the way that you perceive sensations, as well as altering the blood flow around the head. When both happen together a migraine attack develops. Using this model it is possible to start to explain some of the triggers of migraine. Cheese, chocolate and red wine all contain an ingredient which interferes with the chemical balance of the brainstem. Hormones and stress lead to similar effects on these chemicals in the brain. Interestingly, in 1983, a study from Australia showed that an excess of positive ions in the atmosphere may alter the metabolism of the chemical serotonin. Perhaps this gives us a mechanism by which the hot dry winds of some parts of the world cause headaches. The way in which migraine attacks have a particular daily rhythm, occurring most often in the morning, and their triggering by exposure to bright lights, ties in well with what we know about the ways in which serotonin in the brainstem varies throughout the day and in response to light. These situations all raise the amount of serotonin, at least in animals. One might then expect that things which improve migraine, like darkness, or falling asleep, should be associated with a lowering of the amount of brainstem serotonin, and indeed this is exactly what happens. Things which are associated with migraine attacks raise the amount of serotonin, and things which improve or relieve it are associated with a lowering of this chemical. Most of the drugs used in the treatment of migraine have many actions, but they all share the property of being able to correct some of these chemical imbalances in the brain, and in particular of serotonin. There is still a lot of work to be done on this model, and it may need modifications as research continues, but it explains more about migraine than has ever been possible before.

Serotonin is not the only chemical which has been implicated in the causation of migraine. Several others have attracted attention at various times over the last few years. There are two of particular interest, and we shall be concentrating on these. They are chemicals known as noradrenalin (norepinephrine in the United States) and the prostaglandins.

Noradrenalin has often been described as one of the 'stress hormones'. These are the chemicals and hormones which the body releases in response to stress. They originally had a number of important protective functions, allowing the body to put on extra bursts of speed and strength to escape from danger. These days, people are usually unable to dissipate the extra energy released by these hormones, and so they can give rise to a number of physical effects instead. There have been suggestions that the actions of these hormones are responsible for an enormous amount of the ill health that we see in the Western world today, all because most people never learn how to cope with stress. For a long time it was thought that migraine was the result of an exaggerated response to stress and anxiety, and so it seemed logical to try to measure the amounts of these stress hormones in migraine. It was also known that a rare tumour which secretes large amounts of noradrenalin or its chemical partner, adrenalin, usually causes headaches. A theory was developed that migraine might result from the production of large amounts of these hormones.

Noradrenalin causes a constriction of some of the blood vessels around the head, and administering it during a migraine headache does cause a small decrease in the intensity of the pain. If the drug is given to headache sufferers in between attacks, it does not produce either a migrainous aura or a rebound headache when it is stopped. Normally, when blood vessels are constricted for a time, they dilate afterwards. This experiment suggested that migraine headaches are not the result of dilation of blood vessels following a phase of constriction.

Several researchers have examined the metabolism of noradrenalin. It is broken down and excreted in the urine, so these breakdown products were carefully measured. They are indeed elevated during an attack of migraine, but there is no consistent relationship between the amounts produced and the length and severity of the attack. In another experiment, a group of people were examined who routinely woke from sleep with a migraine. In these, continuous measurements of the chemical were made throughout the night. The level of noradrenalin rose over the three hours before the attack started and then gradually fell during the attack, particularly as its intensity faded. Putting these findings together, it seems likely that the rises in the levels of noradrenalin are a result of the bodily stress associated with having a migraine attack. As we have pointed out in earlier sections, the actual attack often starts long before the headache phase develops. Sometimes the body can successfully ward off the attack during this early phase.

The prostaglandins are a group of naturally occurring chemical compounds related to the fats and are made by virtually all the tissues in the body. They have an enormous

91

number of functions in the body and there are many different stimuli which can lead to their production. Most have specific actions at the sites at which they are produced. They are so powerful that the body has developed sophisticated protective mechanisms to break them down as soon as they have done their particular job.

It was first suggested in the mid-1970s that they might have some relationship to migraine. This idea first developed because it was known that giving one particular type of prostaglandin called E1 caused headaches and nausea in many people, and interestingly, the headaches were often preceded by some of the visual symptoms so characteristic of migraine. Infusions of another prostaglandin — I2, or prostacyclin, did not cause these effects. It is obviously important which type of prostaglandin is used in these experiments as they are all very different compounds. It has been shown that the chemical serotonin causes release of at least one prostaglandin in the brain. The migraine-treating drugs ergotamine and methysergide also inhibit the production of prostaglandins in some parts of the body. Several researchers have tried to measure the levels of various prostaglandins during attacks of migraine, so far without finding anything significant. We now know that because of the protective mechanisms which break them down, very few ever escape into the circulation, so these negative results mean very little. Finally, two of the most commonly used and effective drugs in the treatment of migraine attacks — aspirin and mefenemic acid — have effects on the production of prostaglandins. Even paracetamol (acetaminophen) does cause a minor reduction in the amount of prostaglandins produced, amongst its many other actions. The prostaglandins are extremely interesting compounds from the point of view of someone interested in migraine. They do not provide answers to all the problems, largely because some drugs which inhibit their production do nothing for migraine. It seems likely that for a drug to work in migraine it may have to work at several separate points. Just inhibiting prostaglandins is not enough. It is particularly important that some of the prostaglandins and the serotonin system are closely interrelated. The two together may well turn out to be the main culprits in migraine.

The Causes of Headache: The Research Findings

This leads to the question of why some people get migraine after, say, eating certain foods or being subjected to stress. It seems likely that most people can get an attack if they are subjected to enough of the wrong things, but a most important factor is inheritance; a family history of migraine may be obtained in about 60 per cent of all patients who suffer from it, whereas if headache-free people are surveyed, only about 10 per cent of them have a close relative with the condition. Several studies have looked at pairs of twins to try to deduce the influence of inheritance in migraine, but the results have been conflicting. Identical twins have exactly the same genetic make-up, while non-identical twins do not. In most studies the incidence of migraine was shown to be much the same in identical and non-identical twins. So while there is undoubtedly a clear-cut predisposition to migraine which is transmitted from parents to children, this inheritance is obviously far from simple. There is a rare form of migraine in which sufferers have brief episodes of paralysis, and this form is very strongly transmitted in families. It is described as being 'dominantly inherited'. One of the problems which has bedevilled investigations into the genetics of headache is one to which we have alluded already. The majority of people will experience a migraine-like headache if they are subjected to sufficiently strong stimuli, but some people obviously get headaches more readily than others.

From large-scale studies, it has become clear that over 90 per cent of all people with migraine will have had their first attack by the age of 40. There is plenty of evidence that children may already start to experience migraine in the early months of life, and some children who have periodic vomiting and abdominal pains may develop migraine later. It is extremely interesting, and still largely unexplained, that in adults 80 per cent of migraine sufferers are women. In children under the age of 10 about 60 per cent of sufferers are boys. It is very likely that female sex hormones have effects on the metabolism of chemicals in the brain, especially in the area of the pain gate in the brainstem. Recently, it has been shown that there is a strong association between stressful life events and the frequency and severity of migraine; getting married, moving house or changing

93

a job, these are all potent migraine triggers. Perhaps women are caught up in more of these than are men, and this too may contribute to the higher incidence of migraine in women.

Until recently, it was impossible to study the workings of the human brain directly. We have had to rely on indirect markers of brain activity. Within the last two or three years this has begun to change with the use of a remarkable piece of equipment known as a Positron Emission Tomographic scanner. A long name, which is usually shortened to PET scanner. This together with another new technique known as Magnetic Resonance scanning has made it possible for the first time to look at the human brain during a migraine attack. The investigations using these machines are still in their infancy, but they will be able to tell us an enormous amount about headache in the years to come.

Since we have to rely on indirect measures of brain function, what are these? We have used the chemical changes which occur in the body during the headache attack, and we have looked at the behaviour of a remarkable element in the blood known as the platelet. We have countless millions of platelets circulating within us. These have a whole host of functions but one of their most important roles is in the clotting of the blood. It happens that they share many of the chemical characteristics of brain cells; at one time it was thought that they were chemically identical but that is not so, they are just similar. Many pieces of research seemed to indicate that platelets were in some way involved in the genesis of migraine attacks, but it now seems that they have the role of innocent bystanders in migraine. During the attack, there is a state of metabolic chaos. The fatty acids in the blood rise and so do the levels of some hormones. We have already mentioned the rise in noradrenalin which may occur. These changes in metabolism have effects on the platelets which can be easily measured in the laboratory. These changes, and some very subtle chemical abnormalities which are always present in the platelets of the migraine patient, have led us to be able to make deductions about what is going on in the brain itself. One of the most interesting recent discoveries is that the platelets of many of those migraine sufferers who are sensitive to cheese, chocolate, and wine are deficient in a certain chemical, which has the name of 'Phenolsulphotransferase'. This chemical is an enzyme, or biological catalyst, and like all the other thousands of enzymes it exists in nature to control the speed of chemical reactions. This particular enzyme appears to be involved in the removal of a toxic chemical found in these foods. This time the platelet may be telling us something about what is going on in the intestines, but all the other findings seem to be offering clues which lead us back to the brainstem pain gate and the chemical serotonin. We do not yet have any test for migraine to see if someone is liable to get it, but perhaps this will be possible in the future.

In the section on the diagnosis of headache we made the point that tension headache and migraine are different, even though both may occur in the same person. In practice, it is sometimes difficult to tell them apart, even after years of experience. This has led many to wonder whether the two may represent different ends of a spectrum of headache. At one end we have classical migraine, and at the other tension headache. As we have discussed, it is possible to use the platelets in the blood as a partial mirror of things that are going on in the brain. Examining the platelets of tension headache sufferers has shown that they have some of the same abnormalities which are found in migraine. It has also been shown that giving drugs which dilate blood vessels can cause a lessening in the severity of tension headache. Contraction of the muscles of the head and neck, which was thought to be the typical finding in tension head-ache, is also common in migraine. Some people with common migraine can be successfully treated by injecting local anaesthetic into the muscles around the head and neck. Headache from any cause may be associated with contraction of these muscles. It now seems clear that muscle contraction in tension headache is a consequence of the headache, rather than its cause.

So what causes tension headache? The answer to this is not certain, but taking all the facts together it seems likely that it is the result of a constriction in blood vessels supplying the muscles around the head and neck. This constriction may be caused by many different factors but stress, anxiety and depression are the most common.

During the early 1980s, a number of research workers, both in the United States and Great Britain, suggested that many attacks of migraine were caused by problems with the teeth. It was thought that dental problems led to abnormalities in the function of the joint between the jaw and the skull. This is a simple hinge joint which undergoes an enormous amount of stress during a lifetime. It is said there is a high frequency of abnormalities of jaw opening in migraine sufferers. As a result, many patients have been treated with specially designed plates to try to correct the way in which the jaw moves. There have been a number of encouraging reports to suggest that this may be of benefit to a small number of patients. However, when a small scientific study was performed to look into this, using highly sophisticated equipment, it was found that the jaw opening problems were present in only about a quarter of migraine patients. Only one of these patients had any benefit from a dental appliance. This contrasts with some recent extravagant claims that 90 per cent of migraine patients could be cured in this way. The technique must for the time being be regarded as unproven. The best advice is that if you suffer from severe headaches, it is worth having your teeth checked, but only contemplate this form of treatment if it is recommended by your dentist. It must then be done by someone with special training in the technique.

Headache continues to be a scourge for millions of people throughout the world. Research is making great strides, and we can look forward to the day when we can eliminate it from the list of problems facing us. Even before that time arrives, a careful selection of treatments can bring relief to the majority of cases.

Addresses of Self-help and Information Services

The Migraine Trust
45 Great Ormond Street
London WC1N 3HD

British Migraine Association
Evergreen
Ottermead Lane
Ottershaw
Chertsey
Surrey

The National Migraine Foundation
5252 N. Western Avenue
Chicago
Illinois 60625
USA

All the following will be able to answer questions concerning the registration of individual practitioners, and in some cases to recommend a therapist. Organisations marked with an * only list medically qualified practitioners, and will usually only recommend practitioners to members of the medical profession. Your doctor can get information from them if you have difficulty.

* *The Faculty of Homoeopathy*
The Royal London Homoeopathic Hospital
Great Ormond Street
London WC1N 3HR

* *British Medical Acupuncture Society*
67–69 Chancery Lane
London WC2 1AF

British Acupuncture Association
34 Alderney Street
London SW1B 4EU

The College of Traditional Chinese Acupuncture
Tao House
Queensway
Royal Leamington Spa
Warwickshire CV31 3LZ

General Council and Register of Osteopaths
1–4 Suffolk Street
London SW1Y 4HG

British Chiropractors Association
5 First Avenue
Chelmsford
Essex CM1 1RX

Action Against Allergy
Head Office
43 The Downs
London SW20 8HG

Food Allergy Association
9 Mill Lane
Shoreham-by-Sea
West Sussex

* *British Society for Nutritional Medicine*
Dr S. Davies
9 Portland Road
East Grinstead
West Sussex RH19 4EB

* *British Society of Medical and Dental Hypnosis*
42 Links Road
Ashtead
Surrey KT21 2HJ

Yoga Biomedical Trust
PO Box 140
Cambridge

The College of Health
18 Victoria Park Square
London E2 9BR

Addresses of Self-help and Information Services

National Centre for Homoeopathy
1500 Massachusetts Avenue, N.W.
Washington
DC 20005
USA

World Acupuncture Organisation
P Box 722W48
Vancouver
BC
Canada V5Z 2R9

Society for Clinical Ecology
1750 Humboldt Street
Denver
Colorado 80218
USA

Australia

Biofeedback Meditation and Relaxation Centre
165 Adderton Road
Carlingford
NSW 2118

Acupuncture Association of Australia
1 Palmer Street
North Parramatta
NSW 2151

Australian Natural Therapies Association
729 Burwood Road
Hawthorn

Australian Osteopathic Association
71 Collins Street
Melbourne 3000

Australian Chiropractors, Osteopaths and Natural Physicians Association
6/102 Kiribilli Avenue
Kiribilli
NSW

Homoeopathic Association of Australia
7 Hampden Road
Artarmon
NSW 2064

Canada

Canadian Migraine Foundation
390 Brunswick
Ontario M5R 1ZZ

Acupuncture Association of Canada
10 St Mary Street
Toronto
Ontario M4Y 1P9

Federation of Ontario Yoga Teachers
30 Erskine Avenue
Apartment 911
Toronto
Ontario M4P 1Y6

Canadian Society of Homoeopathy
Post Box 4333
Station 'E'
Ottawa
Ontario K1S 5B3

Canadian Osteopathic Association
575 Waterloo Street
London
Ontario
Canada N6B 2R2

Canadian Chiropractice Association
1900 Batview Avenue
Toronto 17
Ontario

South Africa

South African Association of Health Services
PO Box 17055
Groenkloof 0027
Pretoria
(Has details of several available therapies)

Addresses of Self-help and Information Services

South African Homoeopathic Association
PO Box 10255
1570 Strubenvale

Chiropractice Association of South Africa
Poynton House 701
Gardiner Street
4000 Durban

USA

American Guild of Hypnotherapists
7117 Farnam Street
Omaha
Nebraska 68132

Acupuncture International Association
2330 S Brentwood Boulevard
St Louis
MO 63144

National Center for Homeopathy
1500 Massachusetts Avenue, NW
Washington
DC 20005

Further Reading

The following references have been kept brief and are intended to provide background information for the interested reader. To provide an entrée to the research literature for those who wish to pursue any particular points, they are arranged in the order in which particular points appear in the text.

Introduction

Fulder, S., *The Handbook of Complementary Medicine* (London: Coronet Books) 1984.

Chapter One

Dalessio, D. J. (ed.), *Wolff's Headache and Other Head Pains* (Oxford: Oxford University Press) 1980.
Raskin, N. H. and Appenzeller, O., *Headache* (Eastbourne: W. B. Saunders) 1980.
Sachs, O., *Migraine* (London: Faber & Faber) 1970. (An excellent general introduction to the whole subject of headache.)

Chapter Two

The same books referred to in Chapter One contain a wealth of up-to-date information.

Chapter Three

Rippere, V., *The Allergy Problem* (Wellingborough: Thorsons) 1983.
Randolph, T. G. and Moss, R. W., *Allergies* (Wellingborough: Turnstone Press) 1981.
Lessof, M. H. (ed.) *Clinical Reactions to Food* (Chichester: John Wiley) 1983.

Further Reading

Airola, P., *Hypoglycaemia: A Better Approach* (Arizona: Health Plus) 1977.

Lesser, M., *Nutrition and Vitamin Therapy* (New York Grove Press) 1980.

Bland, J., *Hair Tissue Mineral Analysis* (Wellingborough: Thorsons) 1983.

Chapter Five

Anon. *Essentials of Chinese Acupuncture* (Peking: Foreign Language Press) 1980.

Lu Gwei-Djen and Needham, J., *Celestial Lancets* (Cambridge: Cambridge University Press) 1980.

Bischko, J., 'Acupuncture in headache', *Research and Clinical Studies in Headache*, 1978, 5:72–85.

Cheng, A. C. K., 'The treatment of headaches employing acupuncture', *American Journal of Chinese Medicine*, 1975, 3:181–5.

Gwan, K. H., 'Treatment of cluster headache by acupuncture', *American Journal of Chinese Medicine*, 1977, 5:91–4.

Jensen, L. B. and Jensen, S. B., 'Effect of acupuncture on tension headache and urinary catecholamine excretion', *Scandinavian Journal of Dental Research*, 1982, 90:397–403.

Jensen, L. B., Tallgren, A., Troest, T. and Jensen, S. B., 'Effect of acupuncture on myogenic headache', *Scandinavian Journal of Dental Research*, 1977, 85:456–70.

Loh, L., Nathan, P. W., Schott, G. D. and Zilkha, K. J., 'Acupuncture versus medical treatment for migraine and muscle tension headaches', *Journal of Neurology, Neurosurgery and Psychiatry*, 1984, 47: 333–7.

Nemerof, H., 'Acupuncture in the management of headache', *Journal of the American Osteopathic Association*, 1977, 76:699–701.

Okazaki, K., Sadove, M. S., Kim, S. I., Lee, M. H. and Cheng, D., 'Ryodoraku therapy for migraine headache', *American Journal of Chinese Medicine*, 1975, 3:61–70.

Scott, J., 'The diagnosis and treatment of headaches by acupuncture', *Journal of Chinese Medicine*, 1984, 15:5–19.

Chapter Six

Blackie, M. G., *The Challenge of Homoeopathy. The Patient Not the Cure* (London: Unwin Paperbacks) 1984.

Boyd, H. W., *Introduction to Homoeopathic Medicine* (Beaconsfield: Beaconsfield Publishers) 1981.

Weiner, M. and Goss, K., *The Complete Book of Homoeopathy* (London: Bantam Books) 1981.

Cooper, D. J., 'Migraine: A Homoeopathic Approach', *British Homoeopathic Journal*, 1984, 73:1–10.

Chapter Seven

Ambrose, G. and Newbold, G., *A Handbook of Medical Hypnosis* (Eastbourne: Baillière Tindall) 1980.

Anderson, J. A. D., Basker, M. A. and Dalton, R., 'Migraine and hypnotherapy', *International Journal of Clinical and Experimental Hypnosis*, 1975, 23:48–58.

Shaw, H. Laurence, *Hypnosis in Practice* (Eastbourne: Baillière Tindall) 1977.

Waxman, D., *Hypnosis* (London: Allen & Unwin) 1981.

Chapter Eight

Madders, J., *Stress and Relaxation* (London: Martin Dunitz) 1979.

Mason, L. J. *Guide to Stress Reduction* (Culver, Cal., Peace Press) 1980.

Chapter Nine

Barlow, W., *The Alexander Principle* (London: Victor Gollancz) 1973.

Chaitow, L., *Osteopathy: Head-to-Toe Health Through Manipulation* (Wellingborough: Thorsons) 1982.

Stoddard, A., *A Manual of Osteopathic Technique* (London: Hutchinson) 1978.

Scofield, A. G., *Chiropractice* (Wellingborough: Thorsons) 1968.

Kaye, A. and Matchan, D. C., *Reflexology* (Wellingborough: Thorsons) 1978.

Chapter Ten

Raskin, N. H. and Appenzeller, O. *Headache* (Eastbourne: W. B. Saunders) 1980.

Critchley, M. *et al.* (eds), *Advances In Neurology*, Vol. 33. (New York: Raven Press) 1982.

Olesen, J. and Lauritzen, M., 'The role of vasoconstriction in the pathogenesis of migraine', in *The Pharmacological Basis of Migraine Therapy* by Amery, W. K., Van Nueten, J. M. and Wauquier, A. (eds) (Bath: Pitman Publishing) 1984, 149–70.

Further Reading

Blau, J. N., 'Migraine pathogenesis. The neural hypothesis re-examined', *Journal of Neurology, Neurosurgery and Psychiatry*, 1984, 47:437–42.

Wilkinson, M. and Blau, J. N., 'Are classical and common migraine different entities?', *Headache*, 1985, 25:211–12.

Featherstone, H. J., 'Migraine and muscle contraction headaches: a continuum', *Headache*, 1985, 25:194–8.

Johnson, E. S., Kadam, N. P., Hylands, D. M. and Hylands, P. J., 'Efficacy of feverfew as prophylactic treatment of headache', *British Medical Journal*, 1985, 291:569–73.

Steiner, T. J., Joseph, R. and Clifford, R. F., 'Migraine is not a platelet disorder', *Headache*, 1985, 25:434–40.

Index

Hahnemann, Dr Samuel 59, 63
head, pressure points 57
heredity 93
history-taking, homoeopathic
    61–3
hypoglycaemia 37–9

ibuprofen 16
indomethacine 15
induction, hypnotic 73
intradermal testing 35
Iris versicolor 66

jaw abnormalities 96
Jefferson, Thomas 14

Kali Bichromium 67

Lachesis 68
lamb and pear diet 32
'like cures like' 59

Magnetic Resonance scanning 94
massage, Chinese 56
mefenemic acid 17, 92
menopause 14
menstrual cycle 2, 14, 29
meridians 48–9
methysergide 19
metoprolol 18
Midrid 17
migrainous neuralgia *see*
    cluster headaches
Migraleve 16
Migravess 17
milk and dairy products 32
monosodium glutamate 15
moxibustion 54

naproxen 20
Natrum Muriaticum 67
needling sensation 54
niacin 42
nimodipine 20

nitrate additives 15
non-steroidal anti-
    inflammatories 20
noradrenaline 90–1
NSAI *see* non-steroidal
    anti-inflammatories
nuts 32

oral contraception *see*
    contraceptive pill
osteopathy 81–2

pain 86
paracetamol 2, 16, 92
Paramax 17
pears 32
pellagra 42
PET scanner *see* Positron
    Emission Tomographic scanner
pizotifen 19
phenolsulphotransferase 95
placebo response 10, 24, 47
poisonous metals 43
Ponstan 17
Positron Emission Tomographic
    scanner 94
pregnancy 2
preventive treatment 18–20
propanolol 18
prostaglandins 91–2
pulse diagnosis 49
pyridoxine 14

Qi 48

radio-allergoabsorbent
    test 35–6
RAST test *see* radio-allergo
    absorbent test
red wine 15, 27–8
reflexology 83–4
relaxation 78–80
rotation diet 36–7

Also available in Unwin Paperbacks

DEPRESSION
Dr Richard Petty and Dr Tom Sensky

In this book, Dr Richard Petty and Dr Tom Sensky discuss that most intangible of all medical complaints — Depression.

This book is unique in that it was written specifically on the request of those depression sufferers who were keen to learn precisely what happened to them and, in particular, to do what they could to avoid the same thing happening in the future.

Depression discusses the latest research on the causes of depression covering such topics as: genetic factors, chemical imbalances in the brain and 'vulnerability factors'.

With a list of self-help and information services in the final pages, this book is a 'must' for people who either are, or know of, sufferers of this crippling complaint.

THE BOOK OF STRESS SURVIVAL
How to Relax and Live Positively
Alix Kirsta

Stress has become a cliche, a catchphrase synonymous with the 20th century. Stuck in a traffic jam or crammed into a rush hour train, we accept a degree of pressure and tension in our lives that would have been unthinkable 30 years ago. Today stress has replaced infectious disease as the major killer in the industrialised world. Heart disease, cancer, ulcers, depression and arthritis — in all these stress is implicated as the main contributory factor.

The Book of Stress Survival is designed to help you live more intelligently. It adopts an essentially pragmatic approach, showing how to recognise your own stress levels, remove unnecessary tensions, and gear your life to a freer, more untroubled pace. A wide range of relaxation methods allows you to choose a stress-proofing programme to suit your individual needs — from autogenics to massage, meditation to water therapy.

The emphasis of the whole book is on relaxation, personal choice, and finding the time and space to enjoy life to the full.

THE IUD: A WOMAN'S GUIDE
Robert Snowden

Almost everyone, at some time during their adult life, has to deal with the question of contraception. Choosing the most appropriate method of birth control — the method which best suits the lifestyle of the user — can be difficult and confusing. This book will help women, and their partners, make that choice.

* Why choose an IUD?
* Personal factors to consider
* Medical factors to consider
* Having an IUD fitted
* Possible side effects
* The history of the IUD
* Research findings

These are all aspects of an individual's consideration of the IUD, and Robert Snowden provides in this book valuable information for women, and their medical advisers, which will help them make their choice when contemplating the use of the IUD as a means of birth control.

THE FOOD ALLERGY PLAN
*A Working Doctor's Self-Help Guide to
New Medical Discoveries*
Keith Mumby

The Food Allergy Plan takes you, step by step,
through the unmasking of hidden allergies that
may be spoiling your life. A hidden allergy
may be responsible for any number of serious
illnesses — migraine, colitis, asthma, depression,
obesity, dermatitis — as well as a number of
minor complaints such as abdominal bloating,
mouth ulcers, itchy eyes, palpitations, panic
attacks and catarrh.

This remarkable self-help book is designed to
help you track down and uncover the hidden
allergy effect responsible for a sense of ill-being.
The Food Allergy Plan helps you identify and
eliminate those foods from your diet which are
causing you physical distress.

ALLERGIES
. . . what everyone should know
Keith Mumby

Allergies concern everyone. To a greater or lesser extent we are all affected by our diet and the increasingly polluted world in which we live.

Dr Keith Mumby, author of the highly successful *Food Allergy Plan*, has provided in this new book a complete guide to the most up-to-date theories about allergies and their effects. Also, current testing methods are reviewed and sound advice given about how we can all maintain better health.

Based on his extensive experience as a medical practitioner specialising in clinical ecology, and running a busy clinic devoted entirely to allergy treatment, there is much to recommend this excellent guide to the lay and professional reader alike.

CHINESE SOFT EXERCISE
A T'ai Chi Workbook
Paul Crompton

Chinese Soft Exercise provides the new and experienced T'ai Chi student with both the principles of this ancient Chinese art and the benefit of Paul Crompton's long personal experiences of its study and through teaching others.

Unlike previous books on T'ai Chi, *Chinese Soft Exercise* is more than a simplistic how-to guide. Although the reader is given explanations of T'ai Chi exercises and their practice, a wider dimension is created by the author's unique ability to relate this form of exercise to Western daily life.

Excellent photographs by Eamonn McCabe, designed to illustrate the exercises and enhance Paul Crompton's comprehensive text, helps to make *Chinese Soft Exercise* essential reading for every T'ai Chi student, of whatever ability, or practitioner who wishes to increase their potential for a healthy physical and emotional life.

Also available in Unwin Paperbacks